Praise f
Pavel Tsatsouline
and
Russian Kettlebell Training

New Wine, Old Bottles

By Marty Gallagher, *Washingtonpost.com*, Feb 2003

"It's Déjà vu all over again"

All quotes by Yogi Berra

In elite athletic circles the word is spreading as in-the-know Americans are purchasing ancient Russian fitness equipment, resurrecting old exercise philosophies and obtaining significant gains in cardio conditioning, muscle tone and strength as a result. Call it the Slavic Retro Fitness Craze: kettlebells are rustic and raw and are lifted and swung and tossed in specified patterns to produce specific muscular and cardiovascular results. The apparatus has a system, a philosophy of usage, first formulated in Czarist Russia.

Kettlebells have been rediscovered by a new generation of modern athletes seeking ways to gain an edge over the competition. It's at once both a puzzling and predictable reemergence. Kettlebells have pure Slavic origins and have been at the heart and soul of Russian sport-strength training for more than a century. Regular use of heavy kettlebells develops strength with staying power; call it sustained strength. This type strength makes itself available over an extended period of time.

Conventional barbell/dumbbell weight training develops short strength, burst strength: the user hoists maximum poundage for relatively few reps in order to maximally stimulate muscle hypertrophy. Sustained strength is different from short-burst strength. Sustained strength is an athletic attribute particularly prized by wrestlers, boxers, mixed martial artists, football, basketball, hockey and lacrosse players. The common thread is participation in athletic events of long duration where last minute flurries make the difference between winning and losing, between 1st and 8th.

"If you ask me a question I don't know, I'm not going to answer."

Systematic use of K-bells, users contend, provide the elusive athletic attribute of sustained strength. It is one thing to flip over a small car, lift a grand piano or squat 1000-pounds with a burst of short, nasty and brutish (apologies to Thomas Hobbs) power, but it is quite another thing to exert significant strength deep into a lengthy and grueling training session, athletic competition or event.

A lot of men in the NFL might have the ability to bench press 400-pounds at the beginning of a sixty-minute gladiatorial battle but how many could bench that same 400 in the last two minutes after an exhausting game? Sustained strength doesn't just happen, it is nurtured and developed. Through the use of multiple sets conducted with little rest and often high repetitions using exercises with exaggerated range-of-motion, sustained strength is gradually built up, and over time improved and extended. The transition takes time and patience and lots of practice.

Another athletic attribute associated with the regular use of kettlebells is the acquisition of "in-between" strength. Powerlifters, bodybuilders and athletes who train using modern day iron-pumping tactics are tremendously strong within the technical confines and boundaries of the specific exercises they practice, but often brute strength need be administered from an odd angle, a quirky position, a less-than-optimal push or pull position. Kettlebells fill in the gaps and spaces that separate conventional exercises, one from another, and build elusive in-between strength.

Generally speaking conventional weight training exercises can be reduced to two dimensions: either push the resistance away, or conversely, pull the resistance towards the body. Often athletic situations demand the application of strength from poor leverage positions and kettlebells provide applicable muscle power, outside-the-box, filling in the gaps that exist within conventional weight training.

In addition to providing sustained strength and in-between strength, through the use of multiple sets and high repetitions, the Russian fitness system adds a lung-searing, heart-bursting cardiovascular dimension to the workout. This third dimension, cardio intensity, needs to be felt to be truly appreciated. When done on a regular basis (and coordinated with a half-way sensible diet) intense cardio of this type mobilizes trans-fatty acids and oxidizes stored body fat in order to cover caloric shortfall. Determined use of kettlebells burns stored body fat, assuming the eating portion of the fitness equation is kept under control.

No amount of exercise can undo or overcome horrendous eating habits; eat sensibly so as not undo gains. Use of these primitive tools in the appropriate fashion generates an intensity that shocks the user, mentally and physically. Yet results vastly outweigh difficulties and discomfort and the number of converts continues to grow and expand. Introduced to this country less than three years ago, Russian kettlebells have acquired a significant following and garnered respectable market share.

"If you can't imitate him, don't copy him."

The national clearinghouse for all things kettlebell-related is Dragoondoor.com, home base for the innovative Russian émigré' who single-handedly launched the Kettlebell revival in this country, Pavel Tsatsouline. A former Russian Special Forces drill instructor, Tsatsouline earned the prestigious Master of Sport kettlebell classification back in Rodina before relocating from Latvia to Minnesota and eventually to Santa Monica, California. He travels the world introducing and demonstrating kettlebell training techniques, tactics and traditions.

Numerous Police departments and various branches of the Military have engaged Pavel's services and become avid users of kettlebells. Trainees rave over results and share training tips on-line at Dragondoor.com. Pavel runs periodic K-bell certification seminars that are always packed to the rafters. Nothing sells like success and in the world of serious fitness results are the only thing that matter.

The best sales tool imaginable is a human walking billboard, someone who has obtained tangible results using a particular system. Pavel and his business partner John Du Cane have taken the fitness world by storm; like Marshall Zhukov blasting T54 tanks through retreating Panzers at Stalingrad.

Pavel is a lucid spokesman and presents his respective discipline in a concise, no BS-fashion.

"The future ain't what it used to be."

Emanating from Russia, Old School training tactics thought passé are reemerging in an aggressive, unapologetic fashion: this is no nostalgia craze as advocates point to quantifiable results bestowed on all level of diligent practitioners. Kettlebells are round lumps of iron with molded handles. Various poundage kettlebells are hoisted in a wide variety of proscribed moves.

The system straddles two worlds: strength training and cardiovascular training. The system is neither pure strength training nor pure cardiovascular training. Kettlebells stand astride the two worlds, splitting the difference, combining strength training and cardio training. Is this the best of both worlds – or the worst of both worlds? The object of weight training is to trigger muscular hypertrophy. The object of aerobics is to burn fat and increase cardio capacity.

Is it possible to do both at once? Empirical experience of recent years would lead one to say that melding the two disciplines is a bad idea; progressive resistance circuit training was pushed for many years with no discernable results and adherents eventually faded into oblivion. Fitness success is defined as improving muscle mass, reducing body fat, increasing strength and secondarily acquiring endurance, speed, agility and vitality.

Kettlebells stake out the gray zone between the two disciplines. Users handle significant poundage virtually non-stop for the session duration. Workouts are brutal affairs as the athlete tugs, throws, lifts, flings, powers or finesses the bell, singularly, or two at a time, in a wide range of patterned exercises for multiple sets and reps. In a typical progressive resistance exercise the motor-pathway is narrow. When using a progressive resistance machine the groove is narrower yet. A kettlebell uses a broad motor pathway that forces whole series of muscles to work in a coordinated fashion to complete the proscribed exercise. The 'gaps' are attacked and the space between conventional weight training movements are filled in.

With kettlebells, cardio intensity is increased by increasing the poundage, increasing the reps, speeding up the pace and/or extending the session duration. There seems to be little questioning that diligent use of kettlebells can provide a cardio session as intense as a person can stand and muscle hypertrophy will occur if the poundage is sufficient.

"You can observe a lot by watching."

Burnt out? Stagnant? A dose of kettlebell training might be just the thing to jar a complacent body out of a rut. This type training involves a variety of floor to ceiling hoists and pushes; large sweeping movements with relatively light weight that recruit lots of muscle. The muscular 'inroad' is far different than that obtained from the short, controlled stroke of most progressive resistance exercises.

Pavel's classical kettlebell approach favors high sets for moderate reps using a quick pace, heavy poundage and the broadest possible range-of-motion. Pavel's videotapes demonstrate beginner, intermediate and advanced techniques. Seeing Tsatsouline hoist a pair of 70-pound kettlebells overhead in the repetition power snatch reinforces the modern interpretation of that age-old adage: one video is worth a thousand words. Pavel is whippet-strong, explosive power personified.

Watching these videos inspired me to want to test drive this viable fitness alternative. A logical first step for anyone curious and seeking more information would be to pay a visit the Dragondoor.com website. If interest is peaked consider purchasing one of the self-explanatory videotapes.

—**Marty Gallagher**, *Washingtonpost.com*, Feb 2003

"*The Russian Kettlebell Challenge* video isn't your run-of-the-mill advice. Pavel's on-camera presentation is done in an articulate and refreshing manner seldom seen these days. I learned at least a dozen new things. I marveled at the matchless ease he demonstrated while doing many of the one arm lifts. *The Russian Kettlebell Challenge* video is excellent!"
—**Dennis B. Weiss,** author of *Mass!, Raw Muscle & Anabolic Muscle Mass*

"Everybody with an interest in the serious matter of body regulation over a lifetime should commit themselves to Pavel's genre of knowledge and his distinct techniques of writing. Any one of the dozens of suggestions you hit upon will pay for *The Russian Kettlebell Challenge* hundreds of times."
—**Len Schwartz,** author of *Heavyhands: the Ultimate Exercise System and The Heavyhands Walking Book!*

"Kettlebells are unsurpassed as a medium for increasing strength and explosive power. Thanks to Pavel Tsatsouline, I have now rewritten my training program to include kettlebell training, for athletes of all disciplines from Professional Football to Olympic sprinters."
—**Coach John Davies,** Author of *Renegade Training for Football*

"In *The Russian Kettlebell Challenge*, Pavel Tsatsouline presents a masterful treatise on a superb old-time training tool and the unique exercises that yielded true strength and endurance to the rugged pioneers of the iron game. Proven infinitely more efficient than any fancy modern exercise apparatus, the kettlebell via Pavel's recommendations is adaptable to numerous high and low rep schemes to offer any strength athlete, bodybuilder, martial artist, or sports competitor a superior training regimen. As a former International General Secretary of the International All-Round Weightlifting Association, I not only urge all athletes to study Mr. Tsatsouline's book and try these wonderful all-round kettlebell movements, but plan to recommend that many kettlebell lifts again become part of our competitions!"
—**John McKean,** current IAWA world and national middleweight champion

"Pavel introduces the reader to the most effective training tool that most of us had never heard of. I was personally very skeptical about the kettlebell and I waited until I heard others rave about the results that they have achieved with this hunk of cast iron before I purchased this book. Through Pavel's expert guidance (his attention to detail on the execution of the lifts is extraordinary) and the use of the KB, my fitness level has skyrocketed. It is rare to find a workout that will improve your power, strength, strength endurance and cardiovascular functioning but this is what you can expect with KB use.

I have experienced the following benefits from the use of the KB: decreased blood pressure and resting heart rate, greatly improved grip strength and an increase in upper and lower back strength. The most practical benefit that I have noticed is the physical endurance carryover to every day physical activities (moving furniture, mowing the lawn, shoveling snow). I highly recommend the *Russian Kettlebell Challenge* to anyone who would like to move to the next level of physical fitness!"
— **Brad Johnson**, Haysville, KS

"If you're looking for an effective and efficient way to get stronger, leaner, more flexible, and increase your endurance (both muscular and cardiovascular), you won't find anything better than *Pavel's Russian Kettlebell Challenge*. The book clearly illustrates both exercises and routines to get you up to speed.

In six weeks of kettlebell work, I lost an inch off my waist and dropped my heart rate 6 beats per minute, while staying the same weight. I was already working out when I started using kettlebells, so I'm not a novice. There are few ways to lose fat, gain muscle, and improve your cardio fitness all at the same time; I've never seen a better one than this. By simply changing exercises and rest periods—all of which is explained in the book—you can work on just about any attribute you want.

Kettlebells were a favorite tool of the Soviet Special Forces, whom Pavel trained in Russia. He is now training the U.S. Marines and similar organizations with kettlebells here. It's great for martial artists, soldiers, and SWAT teams, but you can adapt it to your needs even if you're a housewife who has never exercised before. As long as you have access to dumbbells, you can do this at home, which is where I do my kettlebell work. Give *The Russian Kettlebell Challenge* a try; you won't be disappointed."
—**Steven Justus**, Westminster, CO

"The most advanced training device is over 100 years old. The kettlebell - the preferred tool of the old-time strongmen - will increase your cardiovascular output and develop strength and endurance like nothing else. The anecdotal evidence, science, and fitness reports outlined in this book will increase your fitness levels no matter where you are today. My resting heart fell from 82 BPM to 62 BPM after only one month of training with the book-recommended exercises."
—**Thomas C. Barrett III**

"I have practiced Kettlebell training for a year and a half. I now have an anatomy chart back and have gotten MUCH stronger."
—**Samantha Mendelson,** Coral Gables, FL

" I would have to say this is one of the most grueling, fun, satisfying workouts I have done. Pavel's books are to the point and I always learn something new when I pick it up to refresh my memory. If you want an excellent heart pounding workout to add to your arsenal of exercise routines this is a must have. I have put my wife through some routines with a Dumbbell and her overall body muscle tone has improved. She says she has never worked so hard before. This not like her aerobics tapes she has been used to. I would say whoever buys the book and goes through the workout will have a very painfully fun experience. Enjoy!"
—**Scott A. Runsvold,** Auburn, WA

"Kettlebells rock. They're one of the premiere tools (along with some well selected old fashioned bodyweight exercises) for developing strength-endurance: that attribute that will allow you to outwill and outlast as your opponents are sucking wind--in almost any sport.
I slashed a minute off of my miles in a month--from 7-minute miles running to 6-minute miles--all without ever strapping on running shoes. Instead I stayed inside with my kettlebell.
And as a special bonus, they're great for fat loss.
At the same time, Pavel introduces strength moves--your pressing strength will definitely increase, along with your all-important "core" strength. In short, kettlebells are a one-stop workout--not something you can say about the treadmill and nautilus health club.
Pavel presents a series of exercises and programs: all of which are brutally effective. Pavel's programs are the most effective that I've tried. Don't be left out."
—**Dan McVicker,** Boulder, CO

"The single greatest workout tool in my arsenal, I mean tools, are my 1 and 1.5 pood kettlebells. I know now that I will never walk into a gym again - who would? It is absolutely amazing how much individual accomplishment can be attained using a kettlebell. Simply fantastic. I would recommend it to anyone at any fitness level, in any sport."
—**William Hevener,** North Cape May, NJ

"It is the most effective training tool I have ever used. I have increased both my speed and endurance, with extra power to boot. It wasn't even a priority, but I lost some bodyfat, which was nice. However, increased athletic performance was my main goal, and this is where the program really shines. Beyond sheer strength, KB's require technique and finesse in order to be efficient. It also builds grip strength, also important in sports.
Where the book excels is in teaching you how to custom design your own program to fit your goals. It is an enjoyable read, and highly informative.
Kettlebells are challenging, fun, and there is no limit to how far they can take you. My fitness has improved greatly and I hope this program can help others as well. Buy the video, buy the book, and buy a Kettlebell. You will enter the elite!"
—**Tyler Hass,** Walla Walla, WA

"In two decades of lifting weights I've never experienced anything like this before. It is incredibly grueling, but the workout really does do everything that Pavel says it does: build explosive strength, burn fat, tone up your muscles (actually more like it turns them to steel). As exhausting as the workouts are, though, and as much as I dread going into the gym most days to do it, it's also surprisingly easy on my back and all the joints that usually ache after a "conventional" lifting workout.

Bottom line is that at a few months shy of 30, after only a few months of the "*Russian Kettlebell Challenge*" I'm heading towards being in far better shape than I ever was in my late teens or early 20s. I'll probably never go back to those outmoded, obsolete 21st century workouts again.

I challenge anyone - who's actually put this book to use - to come forward and honestly say they didn't love the results!"
—**Rob Randhava,** Washington, DC

"Many of the Western basic assumptions about the nature of strength development, muscle flexibility, and even the nature of strength itself are wrong. Pavel's books serve to re-educate us and introduce us to these "new" theories and practices. ...Pavel is the only person who has made these Eastern European "secrets" available to the English speaking world. Yes, his books aren't inexpensive ...But the ideas in those books actually work. The Bottom line: Pavel provides useful information that you won't find anywhere else, in a fun, easy to read format. His workouts can be done at home, they work and they take only 15-20 minutes to complete."
—**David Cooke,** Atlanta, GA

This book is an old, but new approach to physical conditioning based on the official Soviet Army conditioning system by a Russian Special Forces trainer. Kettlebells are different in that they offer a tremendous cardiovascular effect while building strength. They are inexpensive compared to various other systems that offer comparable benefit and can be used in small spaces."
—**Gordon J. Anderson,** Portland, OR

"Kettlebells are without a doubt the most effective strength/endurance conditioning tool out there. I wish I had known about them 15 years ago. I have been using them as described in the book and video "*The Russian Kettlebell Challenge*" and they are transforming me into a superman. It will take some time before I reach superhuman status, because the kettlebells are an awesome piece of equipment. I am humbled by them, but I am also empowered by them. The strength and endurance gains made from kettlebell training carry over into any other athletic pursuit and will give you the upper hand from now on. These are definitely the best tools I've ever used to get functionally fit and strong and I will use them for the rest of my life. Thank you, Comrade Pavel. "You Da Man!"
—**Santiago,** Orlando, FL

The "*Russian Kettlebell Challenge*" companion book and video are well-crafted and user-friendly re-introductions to the lost (in America) art of kettlebell lifting. Pavel and his publisher promote KBs as a tool of "extreme fitness," but the average fitness enthusiast ought not be scared off by the advertising hyperbole. KBs are unique in my experience in combining functional strength and endurance training in a single workout, which you really can do at home. My 4-month experiment with kettlebells has been very rewarding and an awful lot of fun.

RKC (as this book is known among Pavel's "Party" faithful) is the best of his books to date. It describes in words and pictures the how-tos of basic KB moves and variants and gives you the parameters for designing your own workout. While the book and the video can each stand alone, they are designed to work best together. The video augments the book by visually presenting the unusual movements. In RKC, as in all of his books and videos, Pavel teaches his lessons with an appealing sense of humor and a heavy emphasis on safe performance. I started with the smallest KB (about 36 pounds) and found it a little daunting at first. After a few weeks, however, I eagerly moved up to the "medium" bell (about 54 pounds) and now, a few months later, plan to complete my set with the big boy (72 pounds). I am in my late 40's and have been physically active all my adult life in a range of activities, including running and cardio kickboxing when they were trendy, as well as biking, swimming, running, weightlifting, various ball sports, etc. None of those activities has been as much fun, or as productive, as RKC. I highly recommend Pavel's RKC book and video, and kettlebell lifting in general."
—**Gary Karl**, Rochester, NY

"Wow, I have always been a fan of Pavel's books. However, this is his best book yet! I have been doing Kettlebell training for two months and love it. It is one of the best methods to acquire functional strength and is really enjoyable. I can see clearly how it would be beneficial to martial artists and strength athletes such as powerlifters and especially Olympic weightlifters. Pavel goes into great detail regarding the history of Kettlebell training, why they are superior to other methods, and how to get started and progress. Very enjoyable read with excellent photos. No fluff here."
—**Mike Mahler**, Santa Monica, CA

"Once again, Pavel has written a book that should be read by anyone wanting to improve their conditioning. In this book, Pavel explains why kettlebell lifting is such a great tool in developing strength and burning bodyfat. As the book warns: Be careful, this isn't your spinning or aerobic class. Even the lightest kettlebell (16kg) will give a majority of people a rough time at first. You really want to read and then re-read about proper technique. There are a lot of photos to help with proper form. The sample routines give you a variety of workouts from simple to complex, or you can develop your own workout by following Pavel's guidelines. Once you give kettlebells a try, you probably won't want to go back to your standard workout again because they can be addicting!"
—**Steven R Marrell**, Lansing, MI

"I've been working out with weights for over 25 years, and the *Russian Kettlebell Challenge* is simply the best approach I've ever found to combining strength training, endurance, and flexibility. Pavel Tsatsouline has done his usual outstanding job of presenting clear, no-nonsense info on the best way to get into killer shape, with tremendous carryover for virtually any athletic endeavor. The explanations of the why's and how's of kettlebell training are excellent. The exercise descriptions and photos are clear. The training guidelines Pavel presents and the sample programs alone are worth the price of the book. The Russian kettlebell sport standards he includes are inspirational, and great for goal-setters. His "program minimum" can be followed by ANYONE - male or female - in only a few minutes a day, with minimal equipment, and will produce spectacular results. His "program maximum" is a challenge in ever sense of the word, but will definitely get you in the best shape of your life. The companion video for this book is superb as well, and a must for mastering some of the nuances of the unique kettlebell exercises. His kettlebells, which are sold separately, are the coolest toys in my house. I have purchased almost all of Pavel's excellent works, and they have literally changed my life. After years of beating myself up with unproductive exercise routines, I've applied Pavel's Power to the People principles with far better results at 40-plus years of age than I got at 20. Now, I'm addicted to kettlebell training, and more excited and enthusiastic about working out than ever. *The Russian Kettlebell Challenge* is Pavel's best work yet - and that's saying a lot. I highly recommend this book, and all of Pavel's products. If you're serious about exercise and getting into the best shape of your life with surprising ease, you will not be disappointed with this or any of Pavel's products."
—**John Quigley**, Hazleton, PA

"Kettlebell training is hard-core. I have two kettlebells at home, and as exercise devices, they could never be confused with a Stairmaster. They require focus and concentration and are used for demanding lifts such the snatch, the clean and jerk, the bent press, and a whole arsenal of other lifts you aren't going to see in your gym this week. If you've got the focus and can put in the work, kettlebells will yield enormous benefits. Handling their awkward weight while in motion is one of the single best things you can do to make yourself faster, stronger, and, as Pavel would say, more "eeeevil." As a karateka, I have found that kettlebell training has improved my hand speed, foot speed, and striking power, and has made me tougher to hit and tougher to hurt. To my knowledge no other type of training will do that all at once. RKC contains clear instructions and a lot of interesting kettlebell history as well."
—**Robert Lawrence**, Brooklyn, NY

"This is possibly one of the best fitness books I have ever read! I train strictly with Kettlebells and it's taken me to inhuman levels of fitness and strength. Throw off the shackles of easy living and become a living, breathing chunk of steel! Take the *Russian Kettlebell Challenge*; if you're brave enough!"
—**Daniel J. Rodgers**, Moscow, ID

to Julie

FROM RUSSIA WITH TOUGH LOVE

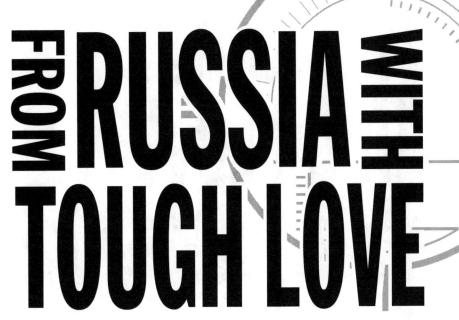

TOUGH LOVE

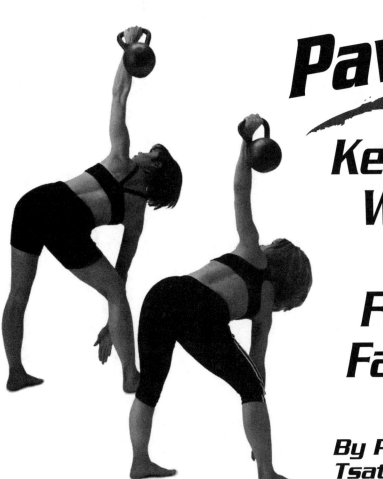

Pavel's

Kettlebell Workout for a Femme Fatale

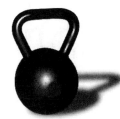

By Pavel Tsatsouline

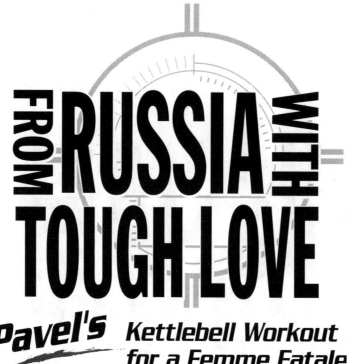

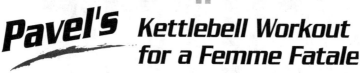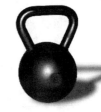

Pavel's Kettlebell Workout
for a Femme Fatale
By Pavel Tsatsouline

Published in the United States by:
Dragon Door Publications, Inc
P.O. Box 4381, St. Paul, MN 55104
Tel: (651) 487-2180 • Fax: (651) 487-3954
Credit card orders: 1-800-899-5111
Email: dragondoor@aol.com • Website: www.dragondoor.com

ISBN: 0-938045-43-1

This edition first published in August 2002

Printed in the United States of America

Book design, Illustrations and cover by Derek Brigham
Website http//www.dbrigham.com
Tel/Fax: (612) 827-3431 • Email: dbrigham@visi.com
Photographs by Don Pitlik: (612) 252-6797

DISCLAIMER

The author and publisher of this material are not responsible in any manner whatsoever for any injury that may occur through following the instructions contained in this material. The activities, physical and otherwise, described herein for informational purposes only, may be too strenuous or dangerous for some people and the reader(s) should consult a physician before engaging in them.

Table of Contents

The Whys

The Hows

The importance of a correct squat and hip thrust…the properly performed standing vertical jump…the crucial distinction between a *straight* back and an *upright* back…tackling the box squat—to improve squatting depth, flexibility, technique, and power.

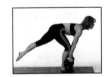

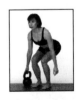

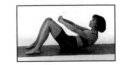

Why the conventional crunch is a waste of time and effort…how to avoid neck problems…the mechanism of *reciprocal inhibition*…the foolishness of high-rep ab training…how to perform Power Breathing for harder abs and a slimmer waist.

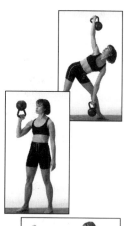

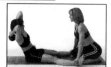
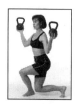

Comrades speak out on the dragondoor.com forum

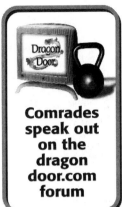

Comrades speak out on the dragon door.com forum

Moscow trusts no tears

Ladies, I train hard men in uniform and do not have the mastery of the women's magazines lingo. I am neither willing nor able to communicate to you on some subliminal level with words like *feel, burn,* and *sexy* or throw images at you of teen models with boob jobs and skin folds duct-taped under their leotards, in the hope you'll buy my product.

Instead, I respectfully appeal to your intelligence. I will present you with a workout that has worked exceptionally well for a great many men and extreme fitness pioneer women such as our models, Andrea Du Cane and D. C. Maxwell. The Russian kettlebell workout is backed up with science, common sense, and a track record.

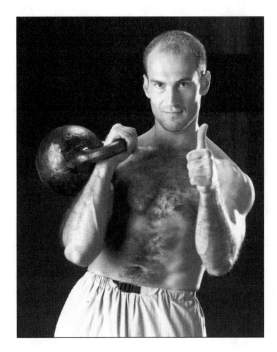

The workouts are brief and results will come amazingly quick if you train hard. I come from a country where there are more female than male doctors and where there are women with thousands of parachute jumps to their credit. I have high expectations for women, and *From Russia with Tough Love*, combined with your will and discipline, will fulfill them.

You are a woman. I want to hear you roar!

Pavel Tsatsouline, Master of Sports
May 2002, Santa Monica, California

How to use this book

The exercises in *From Russia with Tough Love* build on each other like Russian nesting dolls. so please master the moves in the order they are listed. I insist that you observe every fine point of exercise technique. Please read them, reread them, and then review the bullets—or else!

To draw your attention to the 'How's' I have fenced off all the 'Whys' within sidebars. Ditto for the anecdotes and testimonials and the many optional techniques that you do not have to put to immediate use.

You may follow the outlined 4 to 8-week routine to ease into the program. If you have a solid background in fitness, you may accelerate the process. One way or the other, after 2 months, you will be on your own, training freestyle according to a set of flexible guidelines.

Power to you, Comrade Woman!

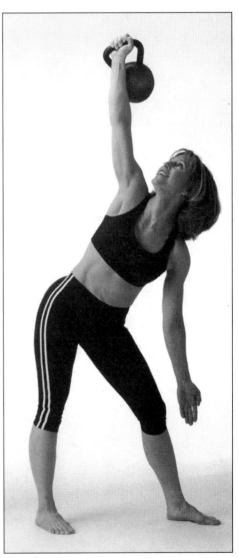

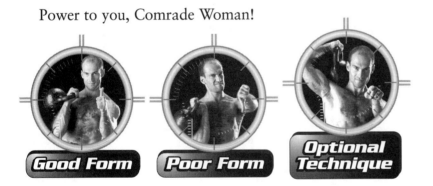

Note: Look for the above icons throughout the book. The majority of the exersices shown by our models show "Good Form," of course. The common "what not to do" mistakes will always be marked with the "Poor Form" icon. And for eager comrades who want more, look for the "Optional Technique" icons. Enjoy!

What is a kettlebell?

A _kettlebell_ is an ancient tool that is going to transform your everyday flabbiness into graceful strength. We could have called our kettlebells _beauty bells_ or something equally gagging, but they were named long before our grandparents were around.

A kettlebell looks like a cannonball with a handle. Apparently, it reminded some strength pioneer of a _kettle_—hence, _kettlebell_. In Russia, a kettlebell is called a _girya_, and I have no idea what that means. Some guys have gotten so attached to their kettlebells that they have named them like pets (no joke). So I do not care if you call it "Cindy" or "Bob"—just lift it!

Traditionally, kettlebell weight is measured in _poods_. One pood equals 16 kilograms (kg), or roughly 36 pounds. Our 1-,1.5-, 2-, and 2.5-pood KBs (36, 53, 72, and 88 pounds, respectively) are cast iron. KBs weighing 0.5. and 0.25 pood (approximately 9 and 18 pounds) have metal handles and cores and are covered with quality rubber-like material.

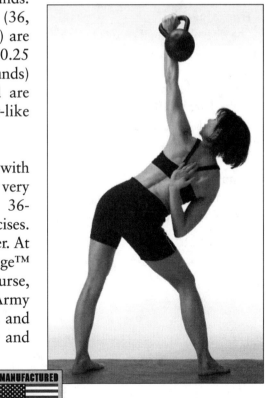

I recommend that you start out with these lighter KBs. When you get very strong, you might advance to a 36-pounder, at least for some exercises. Some superwomen will do even better. At a recent Russian Kettlebell Challenge™ (RKC) instructor certification course, Tonya Ehlebracht, of the U.S. Army Special Forces, confidently pressed and snatched a 53-pounder overhead and humbled many of the men present.

All of our kettlebells are made with pride in the U.S.A.

MANUFACTURED IN AMERICA

Naming Your Kettlebells

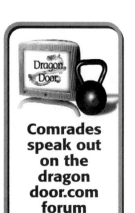

Comrades speak out on the dragon door.com forum

Anyone else named their KBs?
From: Terence

I named my 1 and 1.5 poods "Boris" and "Natasha."

I am saving "Ivan" and "Yuri" for bigger bells. If anyone's bell has a blemish on it, you can go with "Gorby."

The fissionable core of a nuke is called a "Pit". "Pit" n/m
From: Gene

I'm thinking of renaming my kettlebells to "Umph", "Gumph", and "Whumpf".

From: Lemon

…The day Pavel introduced the RKC to us Western mortals was one of the most influential days of my adult life.

My bad. I forgot to warn you!
From: dogchild

She doesn't have a name yet... unless %&*#$! is a name.

Good idea! Mine's named Sveta.
From: CarolynLibrarian

…The half-pood is named Ivana Badasskaya.

From: Steve Maxwell

My wife, D. C., has a lot of names for them, none of which are printable on the forum!

From: cozumelflash

Mine's been dubbed "Bertha." I won't post the name I call her when she is particularly mean to me.

24-kg baby arrived
From: Ogre

Got home from work today to be greeted by my own little 24-kg bundle of joy. Such a cute kettlebell. So I followed what others are doing and named it "Chuck," after a fellow coworker I work out with on occasion. He always manages to kick my butt.

So I told my wife that me and "Chuck" were going out back to play. So much fun! It really is different than a dumbbell. And it makes such a cool impression in the ground when you toss it.

I'm taking "Chuck" to work tomorrow to meet his namesake. I like it.
From: EUR De Molay

Anyone who names their KBs is slightly mad. Then again, you have to be slightly mad to use them in the first place.

What makes the kettlebell special? What is it going to do for me?

There are plenty of reasons to choose the K-bells over the mainstream equipment and methods—or at least to make them the centerpiece of your regimen.

K-bells are a greater challenge than dumbbells and barbells, not even to mention the wussy machines. Try to balance that mean hunk or iron—especially if you tackle the bottoms-up drills!

KBs are suitable for men and women, young and old—as long as they are tough and have no health restrictions.

Giryas are outstanding grip developers, especially if you do plenty of repetition snatches and add the bottoms-up cleans and presses to your regimen.

 "Nobody does it better. Makes me feel sad for the rest." These words from one of the James Bond theme songs might as well have been written about the effect of kettlebells on promoting shoulder and hip flexibility.

They may be uncompromisingly hardcore, but kettlebells are still your best bet against traditional chrome-plated equipment for defining showy muscles.

The KB is a highly effective tool for strengthening the connective tissues, especially in the back. Many bad backs have been fixed with this deceptively crude-looking tool, including the broken back of a man who would become one of the world's strongest. Remember to get your doctor's approval first.

Kettlebells set your fat on fire like no other form of exercise. Losing 1% of bodyfat a week for weeks is not uncommon.

All-around fitness with kettlebells

In the late twentieth century, Soviet science discovered that repetition kettlebell lifting was one of the best tools for all-around physical development. Voropayev (1983) observed two groups of college students over a period of a few years. A standard battery of physical training (PT) tests was used: pullups, standing broad jump, a 100-meter sprint, and a 1-kilometer run. The control group followed the typical university physical education program, which was military oriented and emphasized the exercises just mentioned. The experimental group just lifted kettlebells. And in spite of their lack of practice on the tested drills, the KB group showed better scores on every one of them!

These benefits alone could have easily justified kettlebells' existence—but they were only the beginning. Surprised researchers at the famous Lesgaft Physical Culture Institute in Leningrad (Vinogradov & Lukyanov, 1986) found a very high correlation between the performance in the competition kettlebell lifts, the snatch and the clean-and-jerk, and a great range of dissimilar tests: strength, measured with the three powerlifts and grip strength; strength endurance, measured with pullups and parallel bar dips; general endurance, determined by a 1,000 meter run; and work capacity and balance, measured with special tests!

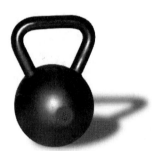

Kettlebells are much less expensive than fancy-schmancy treadmills and home gyms. K-bells are virtually indestructible and take up very little space. More importantly, although many pieces of equipment claim to promote all-around fitness, only K-bells deliver strength, explosiveness, flexibility, endurance, and fat loss all in one tight package—and without the dishonor of dieting and aerobics.

Last but not least, kettlebells, brutish and romantic, are your escape from the dull world of lesser androgynous people into the alternate universe of real women and men who live on the edge.

At last: No compromise total fitness!

KB thoughts
From: Rob Lawrence

The more I do w/KB's, the more I think of abandoning every other form of training. The workouts simultaneously train "everything". Strength, speed, endurance. The thing that's surprised me most is hamstring flexibility from doing one-armed snatches. There is a great deal of truth to the axiom that all training is a matter of trade-offs, but if anything out there threatens that wisdom, it's got to be KBs.

As for abandoning everything else, what's stopping me? Hard to say—maybe habit, maybe a feeling of regret at having worked out other ways for so long, maybe a little voice saying "No, it can't be that simple." But it certainly appears to be.

The kettlebell advantage

Kettlebells RULE!!!
(longish PR ramblings)
From: Matthias

I got my bachelor's degree in kinesiology 4 years ago, and I have been a student of fitness for the past 10. I have long searched for a mode of fitness that could deliver everything I wanted. With thanks to Pavel (and a tip of the hat to Brooks Kubik), I have totally modified the way I look at exercise.

I tried for a long time to make due with cheaper dumbbells, but they DO NOT COMPARE TO KETTLEBELLS. If you aren't sure about laying down the hard-earned cash for a KB, I honestly urge you to make the investment. My dvukhpudovik [a 32-kg kettlebell] has been the best fitness

investment I have ever made, my degree notwithstanding.

And for the first time, I will NOT be sitting down for hours trying to think up the perfect split system or combination of free weights and machines, the best six-meal-per-day nutritional schedules and supplementation schedules, the 100% foolproof set/rep equation, and ROM and time under load. I WILL, however, pick up my kettlebell and just enjoy the pain. And THAT will work.

Re: People of Dragon Door!
From: Rob Lawrence

Kettlebells are better for 200 different reasons, half of which can be explained and half of which have to be experienced. If you don't believe us, fine—that's your prerogative. But I strongly suggest you invest in one kettlebell, and that will settle the matter. I've converted numerous kettlebell skeptics in approximately 5 minutes apiece. As with certain religious conversions, each of these ended with the converted writhing on the ground in agony or ecstasy—it was hard to tell.

People of Dragon Door!
From: Barry1001

There is also a primitive psychological allure, similar to that felt by anyone who loves "iron." There is also an element of doing something that is edgy and that has a component of danger. There are four or five guys on any given day in my gym doing DB [dumbbell] snatches, etc. There is one guy, me, doing KB work. Most of those four or five DB guys clearly want to try the KB; those that have given them a shot are amazed at the difference.

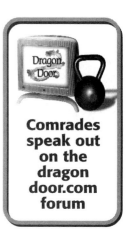

Comrades speak out on the dragon door.com forum

What Makes the Kettlebell Workout Unique?

by Comrade Andrea Du Cane

The kettlebell workout is unique in how it strengthens the stabilizing and supporting muscles. Regular weightlifting actually discourages use of the stabilizing muscles, tendons, and ligaments. The machines isolate one particular muscle group at a time. Weight-lifters are also encouraged to wear weightbelts to support their (weakened) abdominals. What you end up with are big, bulky, pretty muscles that are, for all practical purposes, useless.

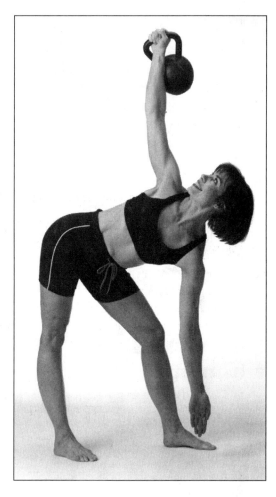

The shape and design of the kettlebell allows more range of motion, ballistic movement, and, within specific exercises, a change in the lever of the weight to the body. By forcing the body to control the weight—without added support or isolating the working muscle—you end up utilizing the deeper, harder-to-work, stabilizing, and supporting muscles. In other words, what you get with a kettlebell workout is functional strength, not bulky, superficial muscles.

As a dancer, martial artist, and Pilates instructor, I see firsthand the value and importance of the deeper stabilizing muscles. They prevent injuries and are essential in functional strength, mobility, and coordination.

Let me give you some examples of the importance of strong stabilizers. First, there is the man who is proud of his six-pack abdominals yet throws his back out when he shovels snow. Why? Because he has weak transversus and oblique abdominals. Another example is the weekend softball player who throws out his shoulder. Again, I'd bet his supporting shoulder muscles, including his lats and serratus, are weak.

The beauty of the kettlebell workout is that it targets all of these important muscles groups in an easy-to-use and relatively quick workout program. It won't add bulk, unless that is your goal. It will burn bodyfat, give beautiful muscle definition, strong tendons and ligaments, and functional strength that you can use in your daily life or other physical activities.

This is the perfect workout for the woman who wants to look lean and have shapely, defined muscles. It's also ideal for someone who doesn't have the time or desire to spend hours at the gym or aerobics studio. The kettlebell workout is great for the longtime athlete, too, who wants to improve his or her strength, coordination, and breath and to prevent injury. And for anyone who has tried every diet and exercise program to lose those last 10 pounds, the kettlebell workout will do it!

How different is *From Russia with Tough Love* from your kettlebell program for men?

The difference is in details. Presuming that most women want to concentrate on their legs more than their upper body—a sensible move athletically, not just cosmetically—From Russia with Tough Love offers a greater variety of leg drills than my book *The Russian Kettlebell Challenge* (or RKC, as it's referred to on the forum), which was aimed mostly at men. At the same time, the arms and chest menus have been streamlined Some extreme moves, which are stunts as much as exercises—the bent press and the two hands anyhow—have been dropped. On the other hand, the RKC book does not have some of the cool moves you are about discover.

Both women and men will benefit from using either or both of the books and tapes.

Can I use a dumbbell instead?

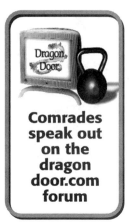

Care and feeding of the 2-pood KB
From: Lemon

Got my 2-pood kettlebell last Friday noon to complete the set. I left it with the two smaller bells to keep it company while I went to work, along with my 35- and 40-pound hex dumbbells and my girlfriend's "Ken and Barbie" color-coded dumbbells. When I got back from work that night, the color-coded dumbbells were gone. I think my large Kettlebell ate them.

My take on DBs vs. KBs
From: ScotPower

Hey! I'm a Scot. Frugality oozes from my very pores. Yeah, kettlebells are kind of expensive. But they will last forever, unless you manage to set off a half-pound of Plastique in your basement/garage/backyard. As for the cost, go find your nearest foundry and have them make you a kettlebell and then get back to us.

I'm sure you can plug dumbbells in for some kettlebell exercises. God knows, I tried. Oh. how I tried. You know what? Trying to use dumbbells instead of kettlebells is like watching a black-and-white filmstrip while your buddy's got the 47-inch digital plasma monitor with surround sound. It just ain't the same, and you will not be able to reap the same kinds of benefits—motor and strength gains—or the same cardio effects, given the awkwardness of high-rep dumbbell "swings."

Re: Dumbbell vs. Kettlebell
From: exrecondoc

YES, the kettlebell is worth it. There is no comparison between the dumbbell and the K-bell. Please reread the last sentence. You will hear that a lot here; it is true. The dumbbell is excellent for many of the drills. The K-bell offers much more than that, though.

Re: Be totally honest with me—KBs or DBs?
From: craigN

KBs are more fun, somewhat safer, and more elegant in the lifting.

Re: KBs or DBs?
From: Rob Lawrence

I just don't think DBs give you the same workout. With KBs, the lifts are through a very long range of motion due to the weight shift. With DBs, the movements are highly abbreviated, especially in something like the clean. I've done the Russian Kettlebell Challenge' (RKC) with DBs a few times when KBs weren't available, and although it was OK, it was kind of unsatisfying.

Re: KBs or DBs?
From: mlilley

I must say KBs add a whole new dimension to aerobic and anaerobic training. Dumbbells do not come close to adding strength to the back, shoulders, forearms, etc. as kettlebells do. It is worth it. You'll be satisfied with your purchase.

Re: KBs or DBs?
From: CoachDavies

I can honestly tell, without reservation, that K-bells are superior to dumbbells.

Re: A question to anyone
From: warnerkallus

The difference is a fine veal parmesano to Chef Boyardee. They are both Italian, but... Well, get the KBs.

From Russia with Tough Love
Basic Training:
Weeks 1-4

Do I need to warm up and stretch before my kettlebell workout?

Static stretching before exercise is a decidedly bad idea. It takes the "oomph" out of your muscles. Just recall how you feel after a yoga class.

Warming up is nothing but a psychological crutch similar to the magic socks a pro athlete "has to wear" to win. Just say no! If you can't, get help.

My friend Dr. Judd Biasiotto is a Renaissance man: a former powerlifting world-record holder, a sports scientist, a Sports Emmy–award winning writer. Read this fascinating account of his extraordinary performance in a powerlifting meet. (Yes, it does relate to the matter at hand.)

"Biasiotto . . . remained fast asleep," wrote a lifter who witnessed Dr. Judd's unorthodox performance. When but five lifters had yet to lift, Biasiotto's coach woke him.

Judd rose, pulled up the straps of his suit, and started wrapping his knees. I had to laugh. How could such a strong athlete be so foolish as to miss his warmups?

"Just another powerlifting moron," I thought. "That's all this clown is."

But when Biasiotto stepped on the platform to attempt his opening lift, my opinion changed drastically. Within less than 10 seconds, he brought about a physiological transformation that could only be described as bizarre. His facial features seemed to change before my eyes. The hair on his arms and legs stood up, and his breathing became deep and rhythmic. His muscles actually seemed to increase in size. The whole scene was a little scary.

Without a single warmup, Biasiotto unracked the weight, descended, and then exploded up with it for a new Georgia State record. The lift was ridiculously easy.

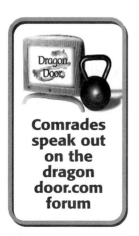

The power of kettlebells

Dragon Door kettlebells
From: Christian Rubio

Mine talk to me, but they are always taunting me. They are never nice. It's only after I defeat them that I feel their power getting sucked into my body. And since they have unlimited power stored inside of them, I get as much as I want out of them. The supply of energy they will give you is also unlimited.

Eight more times during the meet, Biasiotto repeated his astonishing transformation, and eight more times he made seemingly effortless lifts. By the end of the day, Biasiotto had surpassed 10 state records and captured the outstanding lifter's award."

For the record, Judd Biasiotto, Ph.D., did not stop at his state level and proceeded setting four world records. How does a 605-pound squat at 132 pounds of bodyweight move you?! Speaking of strength and no bulk!

To assure the world that he was not one of a kind freak, "Dr. Judd," as he is known to the powerlifting community, conducted a study involving other advanced powerlifters. One group warmed up with lighter weight before performing maximum lifts; the other didn't.

Now, get this. **FIVE OUT OF SIX TIMES THE NON-WARMUP GROUP SHOWED BETTER RESULTS** in the squat and the bench press!

What does this story tell you? There's no evidence that a warmup is going to improve your performance or reduce the possibility of your getting hurt. Even for very big dudes, lifting very, very heavy weights. So don't waste your time riding a bike or doing toe touches, OK?

Just use your common sense. Don't go nuts on an exercise your body is not accustomed to. Carefully ease into your new moves. Start slow and pick up the pace, within a workout and then over weeks and months. Arrange the exercises in the order in which they seem to help, rather than fight, each other. Eventually, once you have adapted to a given drill, you can be more aggressive from the start. You'll have no problem walking up to your kettlebell, cold and in the middle of the day, and snatching it or whatever.

None of this advice is meant to imply that you can never get hurt. It just means you are not any more likely to get hurt. Beware that if you religiously believe that you will get injured unless you warm up, you will. Such are the powers of autosuggestion. So keep warming up and start seeing a therapist.

(You are welcome—for the time I just saved you!)

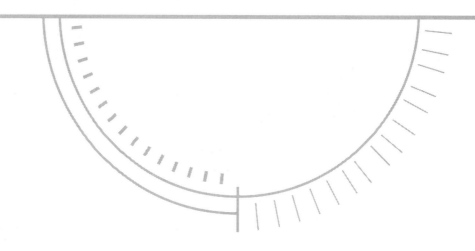

Learn the perfect squat form and unlock the power of your hips with the *BOX SQUAT*

Although our bodies are able to assume a zillion positions, certain movements stand out as fundamental. Take the squat and the hip thrust, for instance. These moves become templates for more complex KB drills down the road and for many of your everyday and athletic activities: picking up heavy objects off the floor, jumping, sprinting, and even punching, kicking, and throwing.

If you don't know how to squat properly, you'll likely hurt your knees or back sooner or later—and not necessarily at the gym. If your body doesn't understand the hip thrust, you're missing out on the tremendous athletic power provided by the strongest muscles in your body—the glutes. Naturally, you cannot expect a hard and shapely stern, either.

To get a quick glimpse of both the squat and the hip thrust, look at the picture of a properly performed standing vertical jump. Note how Comrade D. C. Maxwell starts by rolling back on her heels, pushing her butt back, and loading her hamstrings.

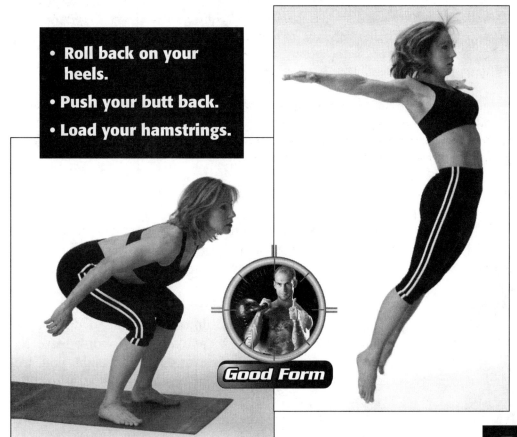

- **Roll back on your heels.**
- **Push your butt back.**
- **Load your hamstrings.**

Good Form

Box Squat

- Forcefully contract your glutes.
- Imagine pinching a coin with your cheeks.
- Drive your hips through.

Note how D. C.'s back arches and then folds over. For some odd reasons (silly and unrealistic OSHA lifting guidelines?), women and men alike shy away from folding over at the hip and miss the distinction between a straight back and an upright back. It's impossible to perform a powerful squat or jump without leaning forward to balance the hips, which are pushing back!

Once in the bottom position, tight and ready to blast off, D. C. drives her hips forward. She accomplishes this by forcefully contracting her glutes—imagine pinching a coin with your cheeks—and driving her hips forward. The weight shifts from her heels to her toes, and the woman goes airborne!

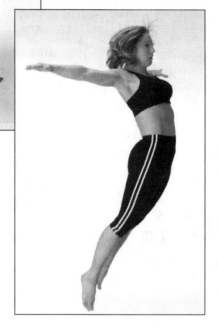

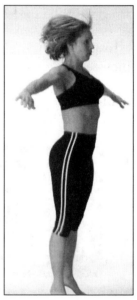

Now, you're ready to tackle the box squat, which is just like sitting down on a chair or a curb. Powerlifters invented this movement to improve their squatting depth, flexibility, technique, and power. It will serve you well.

The box squat groove is almost identical to that of the standing vertical jump, except your heels won't leave the ground. Set up a sturdy elevation at a height you feel comfortable sitting to. (Our models have used an adjustable aerobic step.) Stairsteps might also do the trick, provided they are not too narrow or smooth. So will any sturdy box of appropriate dimensions.

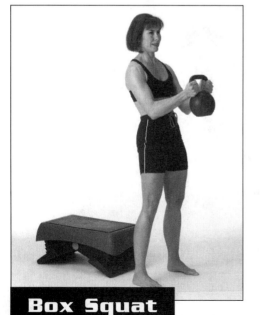

Box Squat

Stand facing away from the step, your calves a foot or so in front of it, and holding a kettlebell in front of you by the horns.

Keeping your weight on your heels, sit back on the box. Your toes may even come off the ground, and your shins will feel tight. Don't let your heels come up, though! If you do, you'll be asking for knee problems and your buns will get no workout.

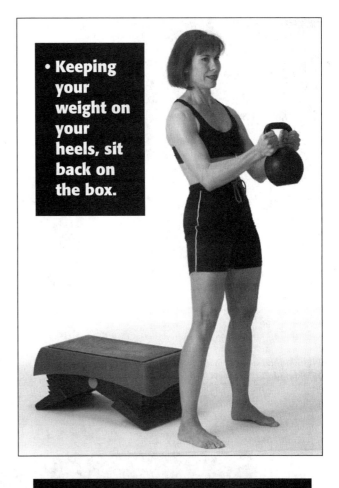

• Keeping your weight on your heels, sit back on the box.

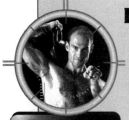

Optional Technique

If you cannot help your heels coming off the floor

Stand on a slightly elevated flat surface(such as 10-pound barbell plates or coffee table books). Plant both of your feet, but let the balls of your feet and your toes hang in the air. Now squat. If you are tempted to shift your weight forward and lift your heels, your toes will dip and touch the ground. This immediate feedback about your wrongdoing will help you get your act together.

• Your toes may come off the ground, but your heels may not.

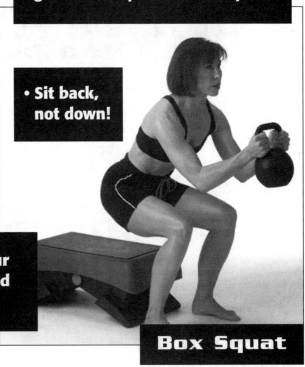

• Sit back, not down!

As shown in the photo, sit back, not down. Arch your lower back, and try to push your butt back as far as possible. Naturally, in order to comply with the laws of physics, you will have to fold forward at the same time or you will make an embarrassing crash landing. Reaching forward with your KB will help keep your balance.

• Arch your lower back, push your butt back as far as possible, and fold forward at the same time.

Box Squat

Never let your knees bow in! Your knees should track your feet, and your feet should point slightly outward.

• Do not let your knees extend beyond your toes. Your shins should be almost vertical.

• If you don't feel your hamstrings tighten up when you descend, you are squatting wrong.

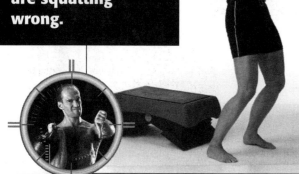

Don't let your knees extend beyond your toes, either. Ideally, your shins should be close to vertical. If you don't feel your hamstrings tighten up when you descend, you are squatting wrong. Imagine that you are wearing ski boots and can't bend your ankles. If you own a pair, why imagine? Wear them for your first few squat sessions! You will have to learn to fold in your hip joints. You will be amazed what this exercise will do for your butt.

Poor Form

• Your knees should track your feet.
• Your feet should point slightly outward.
• Never let your knees bow in!

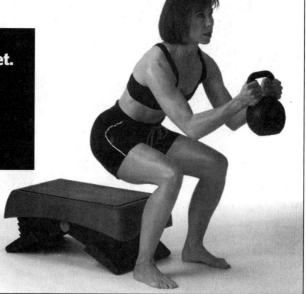

Before you squat, pick a spot on the wall at your eye level and fix your gaze there for the duration of the set. Doing so will help you squat in good form because your body follows your head and your head follows your eyes. (Russians say that the husband is the head of the family, and the wife is the neck.) Looking down will pull you forward on your toes and make you round your back. And looking way up will keep you too upright; your hips will stay underneath you and miss out on all the fun. Looking straight ahead generally helps you keep an even keel.

Box Squat

Keep sitting back until your backside softly touches down on the box. You must not fall, even an inch! Control your descent all the way! If you do flop on the box, you have either picked a squat depth that's too ambitious for you at this point or you have failed to stay tight and balanced. Try again. Insist on reaching back with your butt and reaching forward with the kettlebell.

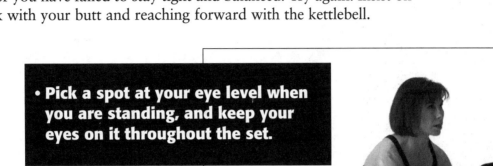

• Pick a spot at your eye level when you are standing, and keep your eyes on it throughout the set.

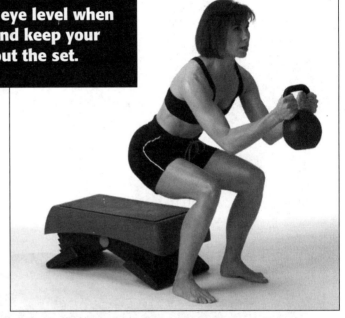

• Softly sit on the box.

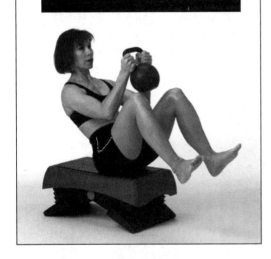

• Don't cross your ankles or push your feet underneath you.

• Plant your feet like you mean it, with your shins almost upright.

Rock back. Then instantly rock forward and stand up while observing the following rules. First, don't cross your ankles or push your feet underneath you. Plant your feet like you mean it, with your shins almost upright. Second, fold over and reach forward. If you have set your feet far enough forward, as instructed, trying to stand up while remaining upright will be an exercise in futility (not to mention a challenge to the fundamental laws of mechanics).

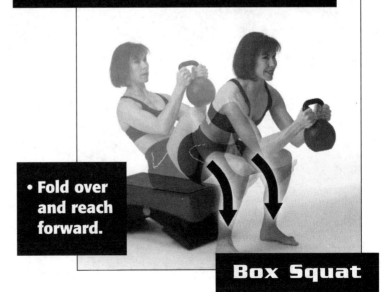

• Fold over and reach forward.

Box Squat

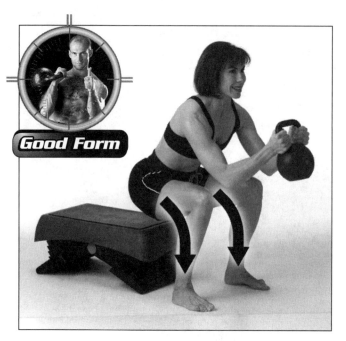

Good Form

The moment you feel that your weight has shifted from your glutes to your feet, push your feet hard straight down into the ground, as shown by the arrows on the photo.

If you are squatting to a fairly low box or your hips are on the heavy side, you will have to hold your kettlebell far in front of you just to get up. It's a matter of balance. Don't lose your momentum, either.

Tense your glutes (remember the coin pinch?), and drive your hips forward until you stand tall. Lock out your knees by pulling up your kneecaps, and lock out your hips by cramping your glutes. Don't even think about scooping forward! Your knees will slip forward only if you completely disregard the instructions to stay on your heels. Don't be afraid to fold over! Drive with your hips, rather than your thighs. If you ignore your orders -drop and give me 10 pushups!

> • **Tense your glutes and drive your hips forward until you stand tall.**
> • **Lock out your knees by pulling up your kneecaps, and lock out your hips by cramping your glutes.**

> • **Don't let your knees slip forward or your heels come off the ground.**

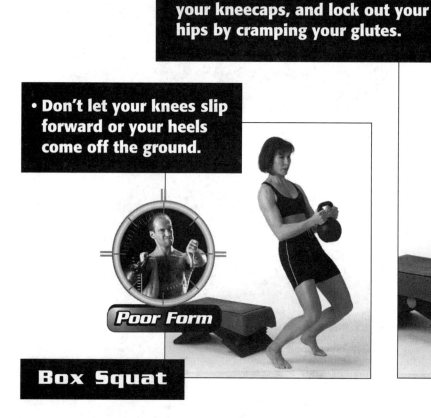

Poor Form

Box Squat

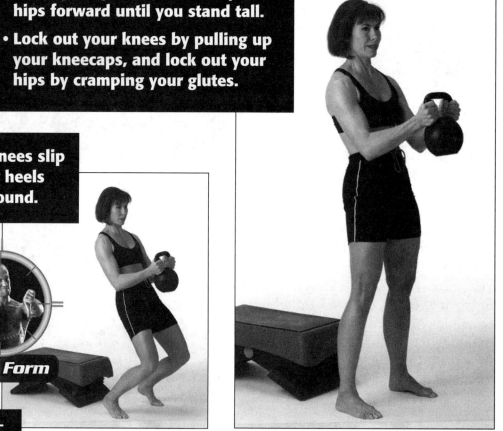

If these instructions on technique for the box squat seem exhaustive, please realize that attention to detail is what makes this or any other program work. Anything worth doing is worth doing right. Besides, most of the remaining drills will build on the foundation of the box squat. So once you get it down pat, learning and mastering the rest will be a piece of cake.

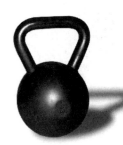

Perform a set of as many reps as you can do with perfect form and control, ideally 10 to 20. Try to somehow synchronize your breathing with the movement.

Do not be a slave to numbers!

Even if your workout lists a RM, or repetition maximum, don't do any more reps than you can manage with crisp perfection. Decide to stop *before* your form deteriorates. And above all, don't become a slave to numbers. Having the mindset of "I did 10 reps last time; therefore, I won't settle for anything less than 11 today" will likely put you on the road to injury, no gains, and frustration.

You can't improve in every workout—at least once you've achieved a decent fitness level, or the point of diminishing returns. If you try to do more, regardless, you will be subconsciously cheating to make the reps. Before you know it, your technique will be atrocious and you'll suffer all the undesirable but inevitable consequences.

Interestingly, while safely lifting with perfect technique builds strength that carries over to all-out efforts with a very heavy weight, bouncing and cheating do not. What you can get away with when you are handling light poundage will not fly once the hard and cold reality of heavy iron sets in.

Take the deadlift, originally called the *dead weight lift*. Basically, it involves bending over and picking up a weight from the floor. The easiest—and the worst!—way to deadlift for reps is to jerk the bell from the floor, with your butt way up in the air, and then bounce the weight off the platform between repetitions. This approach definitely produces the greatest number of reps if a light weight is employed. But after training this way, if you attempt a heavier, low-rep exertion, you will either hurt your back when jerking the poundage off the ground or you will purely fail the lift.

Powerlifters know that a heavy dead must be "squeezed" off the floor and always do so, even with light poundages. It sacrifices their rep count, but they don't care; they know that they are getting stronger, and that's all that matters. Come to think of it, having a near-zero potential for injury is nothing to sneeze at either!

The bottom line: Record your reps, but do not try to top them at any cost. Form and substance over numbers.

Box Squat

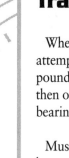

Training to failure—or to success?

When it comes to building strength, the gym wisdom is quick to sum it up as the attempt to do another rep when all your reps have been done and to lift another 5 pounds when all your pounds have been lifted. This "Do as many reps as you can and then one more" mentality of strength development sounds cute and macho, but it has no bearing on reality. It is training to *failure!*

Muscle failure is more than unnecessary—it is counterproductive! Neuroscientists have known for half a century that if you stimulate a neural pathway—say, the squat "groove"—and the outcome is positive, future squatting will be easier, thanks to the so-called *Hebbian rule.* In effect, the "groove" has been "greased." Next time, the same amount of mental effort will result in a heavier squat. This is training to success!

The opposite is also true. If your body fails to perform your brain's command, the "groove" will get "rusty." You will be pushing as hard as usual, but your muscle will contract with less intensity than usual. To paraphrase powerlifting and fitness pioneer Dr. Terry Todd, if you are training to failure, you are training to fail.

Cultivate the "You can't fire me because I quit" attitude. Train to success!

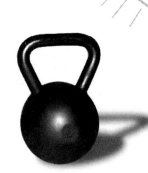

When you're done with your set, walk around a little until your heart rate comes down a little. This practice applies to the rest of the *From Russia with Tough Love* exercises, as well. You see, your heart pumps the blood out, and it's up to your muscles to bring the blood back in. Your veins have one-way valves, and your contracting muscles milk up the used blood back to the heart.

If you suddenly stop vigorous activity, your heart, unaided by the muscle pumps, will have to work extra hard to propel the blood all the way through your body and back. This can be too much for it, especially if you're not in particularly good shape. Walking around, on the other hand, will activate the big blood pumps in your legs and make things easier for your heart. So rest actively!

When you feel halfway recovered—which may happen in 20 seconds or a few minutes, depending on your conditioning—do a set of the special stretches that will be covered in a couple of pages. Then take another brief rest, and do one more set of box squats. Finally, repeat the whole sequence one more time.

After that, feel free to do whatever upper-body work and cardio you have been doing lately and stretch. If you haven't been doing anything, just do squats and stretch. We will add torso and arm work soon enough. And the cardio effects of some of the upcoming drills must be experienced to be believed.

The day after, do two sets of box squats, each with only half the reps you were good for yesterday. For instance, if you squatted 10 and 12 times on Monday, trying hard but not killing yourself, on Tuesday, perform 6 reps and then another 6 after a brief rest. On Wednesday, the party will be over and you will be back to two all-out sets.

"Consistency over intensity" (or the case for easy workouts instead of days off)

Anyone who claims that you can't train a muscle group two days in a row is seriously disturbed. Ditto for the high-intensity cult that denies the value of a light workout.

I can back up these strong words with gold! Hundreds of world champions who speak my native language are the poster children of daily training at varying intensity. You don't really think that Natasha and Boris bring home Olympic medals to Mother Russia after following the health spa dogma of never training the same muscle two days in a row and always allowing complete recovery between workouts?

The neuroscientists never got around to telling the muscle heads that repetitive and reasonably intense stimulation of a motoneuron increases the strength of its synaptic connections and may even form new synapses. This process is called synaptic facilitation. Translated into English, this means that multiple repetitions of an exercise will "grease" its "groove." More "juice" will reach the muscle when you are trying for a personal best. The muscle will contract harder, and you will have a new personal record or 'PR' to brag about.

For years, I have had great success with daily submaximal training, and so did my victims—first in the Soviet Special Forces and later in the U.S. military and law enforcement. My father, Vladimir, a Soviet Army officer, got me started in my early testosterone years. My parents' apartment had a built-in storage space above the kitchen door. (It's a Russian design—you wouldn't understand.) Every time I left the kitchen, I would hang on the ledge and crank out a comfortable set of fingertip pullups. Consequently, my high school pullup tests were a breeze, And later so were my much tougher military tests.

My father, at the age of 65, can do 17 overhand pullups, and he rarely does more than half that number in training. See if your young, studly boyfriend or husband can come even close. And remember that these are full pullups, with the chin above the bar on the top and the elbows locked on the bottom, not the bouncy half-reps you see in gyms these days.

And yes, it works just as well for women. RKC-certified instructor Tonya Ehlebracht of the US Army Special Forces went from doing one to seven pullups in 1 month following the "grease the groove" method. Can conventional training come even close to these results?

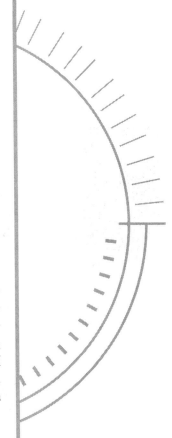

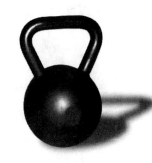

Another reason to have an easy workout on those days when you feel like watching Martha Stewart is what Russian textbooks refer to as the continuity of the training process. Think of it this way: If you include the squat into your leg workout only once in a blue moon, your squatting gains will be nonexistent. Your body doesn't adapt to a stimulus immediately because it doesn't want to go to all the trouble if the stressor turns out to be a fluke. The more often you squat, the stronger you'll get. Eastern European weightlifters squat daily—but rarely to their 700- or 800-pound limit. Constantly exposed to deep knee bends and unable to get out of touch with their purpose, these athletes' legs transform into super squatting machines.

So don't be afraid to have an easy workout or set here and there. It serves a greater purpose than giving you an excuse to go the gym to find a date. As my friend Dr. Jim Wright, senior science editor for one of the Weider Group magazines, put it, the key to progress is "consistency over intensity."

Plus, let's not forget that even the brief effort required to do two 50% intensity sets of squats will spike your growth hormone and your metabolism. And that means you have taken the speed lane to fat loss.

Last but not least, doing an easy session on the day after a hard workout will help you get rid of the soreness. There is no glory in aching, and muscle soreness does nothing to advance your cause of elite fitness. Ask around the gym: You'll meet many women and men who get very sore—and who are stupidly proud of it—yet make no progress.

So take faith! What I'm proposing is not low-intensity overtraining, as your personal trainer might want you believe. It's a kick-butt scientific approach that delivers.

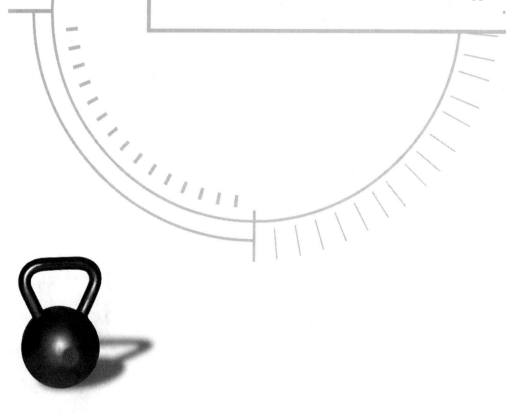

Having said all this, let me show you what your first month of From Russia with Tough Love training will look like. For now, never mind the other exercises listed; just pay attention to the box squats:

From Russia with Tough Love Workouts Weeks 1–4

BASIC TRAINING: WEEK 1

- Sit on a box of a height you are comfortable with. Your knees should not ache after doing squats.
- Add "Good Morning" stretches.
- Start practicing Power Breathing.

Sat
✓ **1 Box squats—2x RM**
(that is, 2 sets of as many reps as you can do in good form)
alternated with 2x5 "Good Morning" stretches.
Power Breathing—5x1

Sun
✓ **2 Box squats—2x1/2 RM**
(1 set of half the reps you did in your recent best set on Day 1)
Power Breathing—5x1   *Plus KB snatch – both hands 14# 15 reps*

Mon
✓ **3 Box squats—2x RM**
alternated with 2x5 "Good Morning" stretches
Power Breathing—10x1   *Plus KB snatch – both hands 14# + 18# 25 reps/each*

Tue
✓ **4 Box squats—2x1/2 RM**
Power Breathing—10x1

Wed
✓ **5 Box squats—2x RM**
alternated with 2x5 "Good Morning" stretches
Power Breathing—10x1   *Plus KB snatch*

Thurs
✓ **6 Box squats—2x1/2 RM**
Power Breathing—5x1   *Plus KB snatch*

Fri
✓ **7 Relax!**

(handwritten: week 3)

BASIC TRAINING: WEEK 2

- Use a lower squat box, but make sure it is well within your ability.
- Replace standing Power Breathing with Power Breathing crunches.

Sat 1 *(handwritten: arm 4x2)* **One-legged deadlifts—3x4 per leg**
(alternate legs after each set)
Box squats—3x RM
Power Breathing crunches—4x4

2 **Box squats—2x1/2 RM**
Power Breathing crunches—2x4

Mon 3 *(handwritten: arm 5x2)* **One-legged deadlifts—3x4 per leg**
Box squats—3x RM
Power Breathing crunches—4x4

(handwritten: Snatch 1x10 18#)

Tues 4 **Box squats—2x1/2 RM**
Power Breathing crunches—2x4

Thurs 5 *(handwritten: arm)* **One-legged deadlifts—3x4 per leg**
Box squats—3x RM
Power Breathing crunches—4x4

6 **Box squats—2x1/2 RM**
Power Breathing crunches—2x4

Wed 7 **Relax!**

(handwritten: week 2)

BASIC TRAINING: WEEK 3

- Switch to an even lower squat box, if you can do it safely.
- Replace one-legged deadlifts with one-arm deadlifts.
- Squeeze a ball or a pair of shoes between your knees during your Power Breathing crunches.

1 **One-arm deadlifts—4x2 per side (alternate sides after each set)**
Box squats—4x RM
Knee-squeeze Power Breathing crunches—4x5

2 **Box squats—2x1/2 RM**
Knee-squeeze Power Breathing crunches—2x5

BASIC TRAINING: WEEK 3

3 One-arm deadlifts—4x2 per side
Box squats—4x RM
Knee-squeeze Power Breathing crunches—4x5

4 Box squats—2x1/2 RM
Knee-squeeze Power Breathing crunches—2x5

5 One-arm deadlifts—4x2 per side
Box squats—4x RM
Knee-squeeze Power Breathing crunches—4x5

6 Box squats—2x1/2 RM
Knee-squeeze Power Breathing crunches—2x5

7 Relax!

BASIC TRAINING: WEEK 4

• Use a box of the same height as last week. No exercises other than the box squats and crunches. This is the unloading week. Enjoy it while it lasts!

1 Box squats—2x RM
Angled Power Breathing crunches—2x3 per side

2 Box squats—2x1/2 RM
Angled Power Breathing crunches—1x3 per side

3 Box squats—2x RM
Angled Power Breathing crunches—2x3 per side

4 Box squats—2x1/2 RM
Angled Power Breathing crunches—1x3 per side

5 Box squats—2x RM
Angled Power Breathing crunches—2x3 per side

6 Box squats—2x1/2 RM
Angled Power Breathing crunches—1x3 per side

7 Relax!

If we look at doing box squats only, a sample first month for a lady in average physical shape might look like this:

From Russia with Tough Love
BOX SQUAT Workout SAMPLE

BOX SQUATS WORKOUT: WEEK 1

• On a box that makes her sit a few inches above the point where her thighs would be parallel to the floor, she would do the following 7-day series:

1	Box squats—2x10, 12	(2x RM)
2	Box squats—2x6	(2x1/2 RM)
3	Box squats—2x15, 15	(2x RM)
4	Box squats—2x8	(2x1/2 RM)
5	Box squats—2x20, 17	(2x RM)
6	Box squats—2x10	(2x1/2 RM)
7	Relax!	

BOX SQUATS WORKOUT: WEEK 2

• Now, on a new, lower box, she would do this series. Her thighs are now parallel to the ground)

1	Box squats—3x14, 14, 12	(3x RM)
2	Box squats—2x7	(2x1/2 RM)
3	Box squats—3x18, 15, 14	(3x RM)
4	Box squats—2x9	(2x1/2 RM)
5	Box squats—3x21, 19, 17	(3x RM)
6	Box squats—2x11	(2x1/2 RM)
7	Relax!	

BOX SQUATS WORKOUT: WEEK 3

• Using a box that makes her thighs go below parallel:

1	Box squats—4x12, 11, 10, 8	(4x RM)
2	Box squats—2x6	(2x1/2 RM)
3	Box squats—4x14, 12, 9, 9	(4x RM)
4	Box squats—2x7	(2x1/2 RM)
5	Box squats—4x15, 12, 11, 9	(4x RM)
6	Box squats—2x8	(2x1/2 RM)
7	Relax!	

BASIC TRAINING: WEEK 3

• Using the same height box as the last week, she goes below parallel again.

1	Box squats—2x18, 16, 15	(2x RM)
2	Box squats—2x9	(2x1/2 RM)
3	Box squats—2x22, 19, 19	(2x RM)
4	Box squats—2x11	(2x1/2 RM)
5	Box squats—2x24, 21, 19	(2x RM)
6	Box squats—2x12	(2x1/2 RM)
7	Relax!	

Interesting, isn't it? You add sets in Weeks 2 and 3 while increasing the squat depth at the same time. Both your training volume and intensity increase. You are easing your muscles, joints, ligaments, and the rest of your system into the program of *From Russia with Tough Love*. Your bodyfat is starting to melt away, and you have more than a hint of muscle tone in your hips and thighs. You are feeling fine!

By the end of the Week 3, you might still feel on top of the world, but chances are, you will be a little tired. Either way, in the Week 4, you don't have to go any deeper and you get to cut your sets in half! When the month is up, your strength and tone will amaze you, and you will feel fresh as a cucumber. (Russians have a thing against daisies—you wouldn't understand.)

Delayed adaptation (or taking it easy for greater gains)

A Russian anecdote tells about a giraffe who laughs at a joke three times: the first time because everyone laughs, the second time because he finally gets it, and the third time because he realizes he didn't get it in the first place.

Every living organism is a proverbial giraffe: It responds to any stressor with a lag. For example, the once popular Rotation Diet does its job by reducing the calories for a day or two and then bringing them back up. A couple of pounds can be knocked off before the slow-to-respond BMR has time to adjust downward.

Renegade Russian scientist Professor Vladimir Zatsiorsky explains this *delayed training effect:*

During periods of strenuous training, athletes cannot achieve the best performance results for two main reasons. First, it takes time to adapt to the training stimulus. Second, hard training work induces fatigue that accumulates over time. So a period of relatively easy exercise is needed to realize the effect of the previous hard sessions—to reveal the delayed training effect. Adaptation occurs mainly when a retaining or detraining load is used after a stimulating load.

The adaptation lag has a tremendous impact on your fitness training. Once you appreciate its power, you'll be free of the near-religious fear of overtraining that plagues the programs found in most gyms. Indeed, intelligent short-term overtraining is one of the most powerful tools in the fitness arsenal!

Many of the complex tapering systems out there would put a Ph.D. to sleep. Fortunately, you can make great gains while keeping things very simple. Just follow the no-brainer cycling procedure recommended by Russian coach and author Leonid Ostapenko: "A very simple method is quite acceptable: after three weeks of powerful, shock overloads spend one week training with half the sets in every exercise."

Stretch and strengthen your glutes and hamstrings with the "GOOD MORNING" stretch

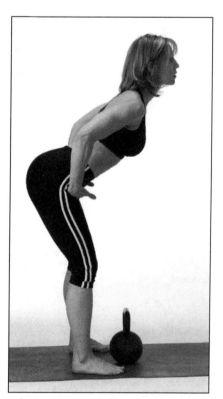

Good Morning

The "Good Morning" stretch, an exercise in precision, will further tone and strengthen your hips and make them more flexible. It will also improve your squatting depth and technique. Add the "Good Morning" stretch to your regimen on the very first day you're on the program. But before doing it with a kettlebell, get into the groove without using a weight.

Rock back on your heels, your knees slightly bent, and push your butt back. Stick the ridges of your hands into the creases where your thighs meet your torso. (This is a tip from RKC-certified instructor Kathy Foss Bakkum.)

Keep pressing your hands in, and keep pushing your butt back. Arch your back tight. Your ribcage must be forced open, and your eyes should fix on a spot straight ahead.

When your hamstrings tighten up and stop your descent, squeeze your glutes and straighten out.

How to get very strong without bulking up

A legend of the iron game, Russian weightlifting champion Yuri Vlasov (the new wording implies that he is a Russian national champion but he is a world champion), quipped that judging one's strength by his or her size was akin to judging a book by its thickness. In fact, it's not the beef but a superior *mind-muscle link* that enables lightweight-class strength athletes of both sexes to excel.

There are two ways to increase strength: structural and functional. The *structural approach* to strength training increases the muscle mass. A larger muscle may be compared to an engine with more cylinders. It's more powerful.

But developing strength through building muscle mass does not appeal to most women. I understand that. And so there's the *functional approach*, which increases strength by making better use of the existing muscle mass. It's estimated that the average person uses only a fraction of the strength his or her muscles are capable of. Using the same car engine analogy, most people are firing only two or three of their eight cylinders. By activating more of your muscle "cylinders" *(recruitment)* and "firing" them at a greater frequency *(firing rate)*, or learning to contract your muscles harder, you will build strength without adding extra muscle.

Remember this equation: **Tension = Force.** The more your muscles tense, the greater strength they display. Force and tension are essentially the same thing. That's why functional strength training can be summed up as "acquiring the skill to generate more tension."

To acquire a skill takes *practice*. So don't think you're going to gain any strength by barely going through the motions of a strength exercise. You shouldn't *mindlessly* 'work out' your muscles, but rather consciously practice maximally tensing them in the context of your *From Russia with Tough Love* exercises.

Now, back to your exercises. Do the same thing with a kettlebell. Safely pick up a KB from the floor by its handle using two hands. Inhale, open your chest, rock back on your heels, and push your butt back. Again, keep your back arched and fold at the hips. As with box squats, don't go straight down! And don't bend over with a humped over back, either!

- **Safely pick up a KB from the floor by its handle using two hands.**

- **Safely pick up a KB from the floor by its handle using two hands.**
- **Inhale, open your chest, rock back on your heels, and push your butt back.**

- **Fold at the hips.**

- **Keep your back arched.**

Your toes may come off the floor (your shin muscles will contract) but never your heels. When your tensing hams make it impossible for you to go deeper while keeping good form, release your breath with a sigh of relief. You will immediately sink a little deeper. (This cool phenomenon is explained in my book *Relax into Stretch*.) Still don't let your back round! It's not easy—but then, if it was, everyone would be doing it.

Inhale, squeeze your cheeks, and straighten out. You should feel your heels digging hard into the floor and your glutes nearly cramping on the ride up.

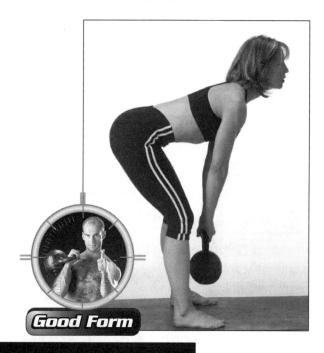

Good Form

Good Morning

- **When your tensing hams make it impossible to go deeper in good form, release your breath with a sigh of relief.**
- **Sink a little deeper on the exhalation; never let your back round.**
- **Inhale, contract your glutes, and straighten out.**

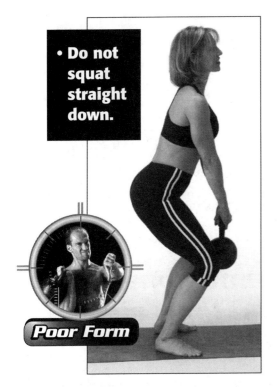

• Do not squat straight down.

Poor Form

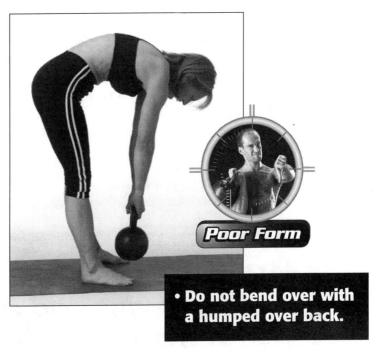

Poor Form

• Do not bend over with a humped over back.

Repeat this exercise 5 times, emphasizing flexibility and total control. We keep the "Good Morning" stretch reps low to assure focused performance and back safety.

On the heavy days in Week 1, perform 2 sets, alternating with the box squats: that is, a set of box squats, a minute or so of rest, a set of 5 "Good Morning" stretches, a set of box squats, a minute or so of rest, a set of 5 "Good Morning" stretches.

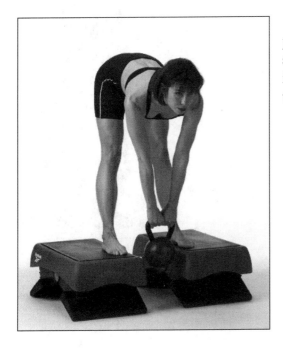

If you are flexible enough, you may practice your "Good Morning" stretches on an elevation. Don't forget that your back is not supposed to round.

Good Morning

What is muscle tone, and how do I get it?

Flex your biceps the way boys do when they show off. Wow, the little ball is just rippling under your skin! If you don't feel like walking around and flexing all day, you could just train your nervous system to keep your muscles taught when you are relaxed. After all, that's what muscle tone is: residual tension in a relaxed muscle!

Strength = Tension = Tone. It's that simple. Generally, the stronger you are, the harder you will be—provided that you gain strength by learning to generate tension, rather than by building muscle. Strength and tone training are the same thing.

Blast your glutes, hams, inner and outer thighs and even your abs with the ONE-LEGGED DEADLIFT

You will be shocked by the quick improvement you see in your muscle tone and strength with this old-time favorite! Besides, the one-legged deadlift will teach you the very valuable skill of staying tight, which is essential for safety and performance.

Park two kettlebells side by side, but give your foot enough room to fit in between them. Fold over at your hips, semisquat, and grab the K-belles. Your body alignment should be identical to that of the box squats and the "Good Morning" stretches: You have more weight on your heel than your toes, your back is straight but not upright, your knees are not slipping forward, your eyes are looking straight ahead, and so on. (I will not repeat myself again!)

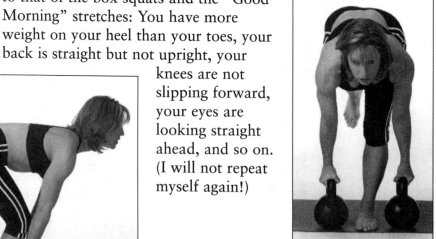

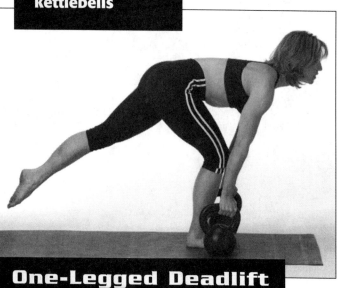

• **Give your foot enough room to fit in between the kettlebells**

One-Legged Deadlift

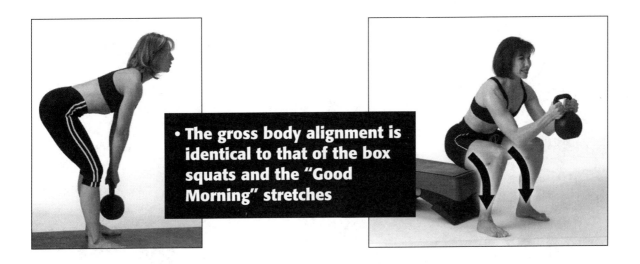

• The gross body alignment is identical to that of the box squats and the "Good Morning" stretches

See how Comrade D. C. lifts her other leg behind her, takes a normal breath into her stomach, and stands up with complete control?

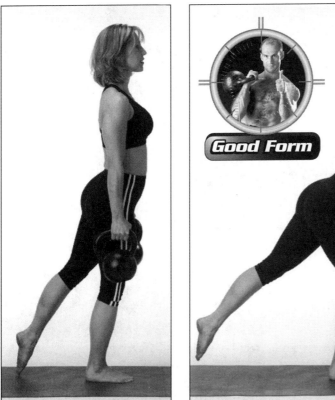

Good Form

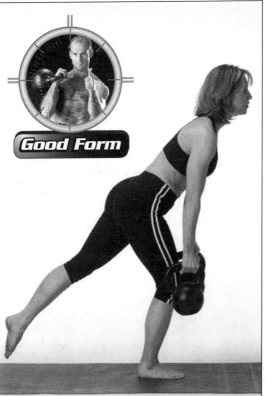

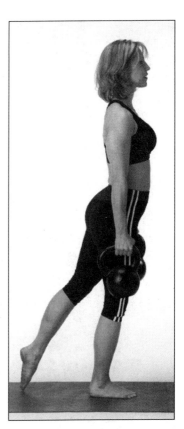

And she does all this without getting crooked!

One-Legged Deadlift

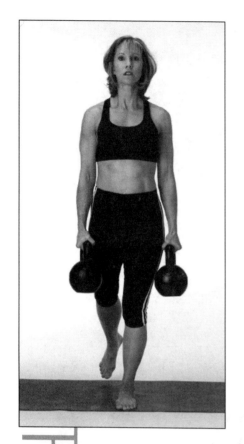

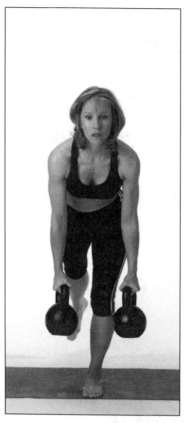

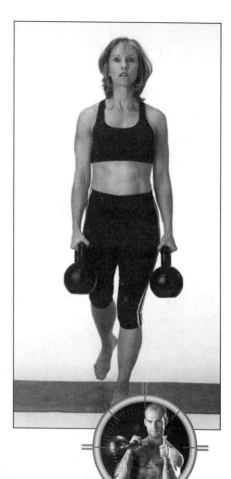

Good Form

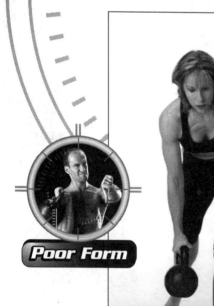

• Don't allow the body to get crooked

Poor Form

Warning!

If you have high blood pressure, a heart condition, or other health concerns, do not hold your breath or employ the high-pressure breathing techniques described further in this book during this or any other exercise. Always consult with your physician.

One-Legged Deadlift

Is it bad to hold your breath?

To clear the air on this subject, let me refer to the world's leading sports scientists, Professors Verkhoshansky and Siff, the authors of *Supertraining.*:

Many medical and other authorities state that one should never hold the breath when training with weights. This well-meaning, but misinformed, advice can lead to serious injury. . . . The breath-holding (or Valsalva) maneuver increases the pressure in your abdomen and supports your lower spine. Without breath-holding, far greater pressure is exerted on vulnerable structures of the lumbar spine, in particular the intervertebral disks and ligaments. Prolonged breath-holding (of more than a few seconds) causes a dramatic increase in blood-pressure, followed by a sudden drop in this pressure after exhalation, so it is definitely not advisable to anyone, particularly older folk and those with cardiovascular disease.

And according to Drs. Stone and O'Bryant, "Damage to the normal cardiovascular system [from straining during breath-holding] is at best rare if not nonexistent." Comrades who have a preexisting condition could indeed bite the big one. Even if you are perfectly healthy, discuss this murky business with your physician.

But don't try it on your own yet; practice without kettlebells first. You will notice that balance is very tricky. Here's what you should do: First, grip the ground with your toes. (Note that our models are barefoot; it's a healthier and more natural way to workout. "Me Tarzan; you Jane.")

Second, tense the glute of the loaded leg. Third, pull the inner-thigh muscles of the same leg up into your groin. Fourth, tense your abs. (Tensing your abs doesn't mean sucking them in to impress somebody or sticking them out. Just brace for an imaginary punch.)

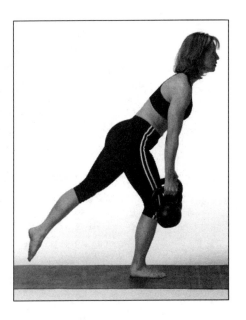

Next, push straight down with your leg and "squeeze" the bells off the ground—or off an elevation, if you don't feel ready to pull from the floor—all the while maintaining whole-body tightness. If you start to lose your balance, briefly touch down with your airborne leg until you get it back. Otherwise, maintain your balance by staying tight—like a ballet dancer or a gymnast— rather than swaying around. It's a good idea to have a spotter around in the beginning. Be very careful with your knee; don't wrench it by thrashing around!

One-Legged Deadlift

Now straighten out. It's essential that you drive your hips forward by contracting your glutes and lock out your knee by pulling up your kneecap at the top of the deadlift.

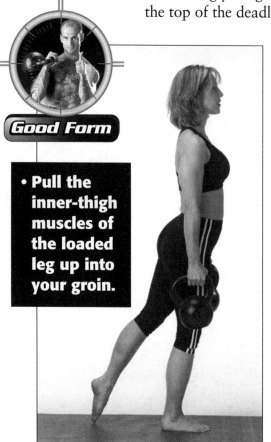

Good Form

- **Pull the inner-thigh muscles of the loaded leg up into your groin.**

- **Grip the ground with your toes.**
- **Tense the glute of your loaded leg.**
- **Tense your abs by bracing for an imaginary punch.**
- **Push straight down with your leg and "squeeze" the bells off the ground while maintaining whole-body tightness,**
- **Maintain your balance by staying tight rather than swaying around.**
- **If you lose your balance, briefly touch down with your airborne leg until you get it back.**
- **Don't wrench your knee by thrashing about!**
- **Straighten out and drive your hips forward by contracting your glutes.**
- **Lock out your knee by pulling up your kneecap on the top of the deadlift.**

Catch your breath and head down to the floor, breathing (or not breathing) as you find comfortable. Don't just bend forward but crease at your hips as if you're doing the "Good Morning" stretch. Let your K-bells rest on the ground for a moment. Tense your body again and repeat.

- **Don't just bend forward but crease at your hips as if you're doing the "Good Morning" stretch.**
- **Let your K-bells rest on the ground for a moment; tense your body again and repeat.**

You may also do the drill with a single kettlebell, but you will have to pay extra care to protect your back, as the bell will have to be more in front of you. Lifting your free leg higher —think arabesque!—and keeping your stomach tight should do the job.

By the way, the one-legged deadlift does a fine job of strengthening your ankles—at least if you lift barefoot, as instructed. An average weak ankle tends

One-Legged Deadlift

Protect your back with tight abs

Instant back pain cure!
From: Comrade Yuri

I was a real klutz and fell back right onto my tailbone. I felt the kind of snap you feel when you lift improperly and was flooded with lower-back pain. Then I remembered what Andy68 said he was doing for back pain (Thanks, Andy!) and decided to give it a try. I stood up—not an easy task—and flexed my abs as hard as I could. Then I clenched my glutes for all I was worth. After about 5 minutes, the back pain was totally gone. I consciously kept my abs tight all day, and by the end of the day, I was cleaning the 2-pood with no back pain whatsoever. The next day, I cleaned and snatched the 2-pood with no problem. Comrades, PTP [Power to the People!] is not rocket science . It's better! Power to the people!

Another "What the heck" effect, and it's long, so don't read it if you don't want to
From: Medic1

OK, been hitting the K-bells with a vengeance as hard as I safely can. Well, today I got some proof. My wife and I ordered a king-sized bed, and it finally came in today. No problem, except that we live four flights up! Two guys showed up to deliver the bed. Me being me, I jumps in and takes on my fair share. The stairwell is really tight, so we had to slide it up the banister at times. We were just about to make the final turn when something went wrong and the whole thing started going over the banister. Now, for as long as my loving wife has been waiting for this bed, I was fully prepared to sail right over the banister with it in the hopes that the body cast I would probably be in next time I saw her would get me a few sympathy points. Otherwise, she would just say, "Why didn't you try to catch it" and I would be in the doghouse. I grabbed the box it was in and latched down for all I was worth (K-bell forearms!!!). By reflex, I locked down my abs and tightened every muscle in my body. This move alone is probably the ONLY reason I didn't throw out my back. After a few seconds of "Oh my God, I can't believe I caught it!" I wrestled it back onto the banister and up the stairs. THANK YOU PAVEL!!!!!!! Not only am I stronger, but I'm lifting (and not just weights) SMARTER!!!

Remember to keep the abdominal pressure high
From: DaveBrown

I remember the abdominal tension—my bad back loves it! I can't tell how many times yesterday—when I had to pick something up, help the kids with something, etc.—I thought "Wait, tense those abs nice and tight." My back was pleased!

Dragon Door

Comrades speak out on the dragon door.com forum

to buckle in when the person is standing on one foot, especially with an extra weight. The movement of the sole of the foot outward is called eversion. Under the circumstances, it's bad news for your leg. A barefoot one-legged deadlift will strengthen those muscles on the inside of the lower leg that are responsible for inversion, or drawing the sole inward. Just grip the ground hard with your toes, keep the muscles around your ankle and on the bottom of your foot rigid, and make sure that the inside of your paw does not come down to the floor. You should feel pressure on the outer edge of your foot.

One-Legged Deadlift

I believe that you will be pleased with the tight feeling all over your legs following this exercise. The one-legged dead will replace the "Good Morning" stretch in Week 2. In addition to its strength- and tone-promoting benefits, this drill will teach you to stay tight for other From Russia with Tough Love exercises.

Note that you will be doing only 3 sets of 4 repetitions per leg, even though you might be good for a lot more reps. The idea is to enable you to generate the greatest tension in your muscles and focus on your form. You also do these before the box squats because you will be too tired after the squats to have a great one-leg deadlift technique, at least this early in the game.

Strengthen and harden your whole body (and especially your obliques) with the ONE-ARM DEADLIFT

In Week 3, you will keep squatting, but the one-legged deadlift, which must have become your favorite, will be dropped in favor of another deadlift: the one arm. You must pay 100% attention to what's going on in your body. The purpose of doing the new moves is not just strengthening and toning but also teaching the valuable skill of keeping your whole body tight, strong, and well protected in any exertion—in and out of the gym.

Lifting the weight vs. feeling the muscle vs. feeling the muscleS

There are two types of focus in resistance training: external and internal. Having *external focus* means you're thinking of little else but lifting the weight—somehow, anyhow. When a teenage boy is trying to impress the girls with his benchpress and elevates the barbell with atrocious form (he will miss his shoulders when they're gone), he is externally focusing. No comment is necessary; you will reap only an illusion of strength and a lifetime of pain.

In a conversation with a Super Slow™ guru Ken Hutchins his associate Keith Johnson, M.D., coined the word internalization for concentrating on the *process* of lifting the weight instead of the results:

One-Arm Deadlift

They urge you to beat the equipment. As . . . a competitor you must defeat. They teach you to externalize a feigned aggression. You do the opposite. You seem to advocate reaching inside your body. When exercising he [Hutchins's subject] seems to turn off his surrounding environment and concentrate into an internalized trance. That's the fitting word: "'internalize."

Don't interpret these remarks as an endorsement of the Super Slow™ system but do yourself a favor and recognize the point that's being made.

And then go a step beyond. "Feeling the muscle" traditionally means trying to *isolate* the primary working muscle while trying very hard to *relax* the rest of the body. A bad idea.

Strength-training authority Dr. Ken Leistner once quipped that a body molded with a number of isolation exercises, like leg extensions or triceps kickbacks, looked like "a collection of body parts." It just lacks grace, power, and flow. A gymnast, a martial artist, or a ballet dancer, whose panther-like lines you admire, *never* isolates. In fact, he or she *integrates*.

Watch the amazing stunts of the acrobats of the Cirque du Soleil. You won't see sagging bodies with isolated muscles but long and taught entities. Expert performers use full-body tension to channel their energy into the primary muscles responsible for the job. So feel all your muscles, not just one.

Wise old people can tell you that finding a way to enjoy the process, instead of focusing on the outcome, always brings better results than grinding your teeth, aiming for the stars, and quitting halfway through. Commit to terminating your sets a rep or two short of failure and tackle your weights with Swiss-watch precision. If you do, heavy metal will become your best friend, and strength will be your reward.

Assume the now-familiar "ready" position for a standing vertical jump, your hand gripping a kettlebell right outside your foot. Take a normal breath into your belly, tighten up your whole body, and "squeeze" the bell off the ground.

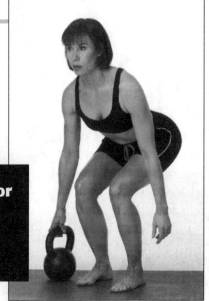

• Assume the "ready" position for a standing vertical jump, your hand gripping a kettlebell just outside your foot.

One-Arm Deadlift

Very important: This is not a side bend! Don't let one side of your body come up before the other! Imagine that you have a kettlebell of the same weight in your other hand. If you own two kettlebells of the same size, you may stand in the middle and alternate arms with each new rep.

- Take a normal breath into your belly, tighten up your whole body, and "squeeze" the bell off the ground.
- Keep your core very tight. Focus especially on your oblique and glute on the side opposite the kettlebell.

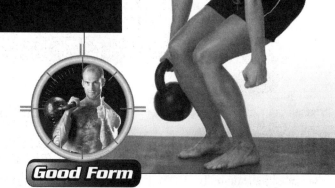

Good Form

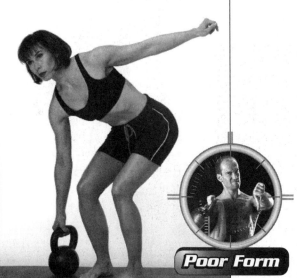

Poor Form

- This is not a side bend. Don't let one side of your body come up before the other! Imagine that you have a kettlebell of the same weight in your other hand.

- If you own two kettlebells of the same size, you may stand in the middle and alternate arms with each new rep.

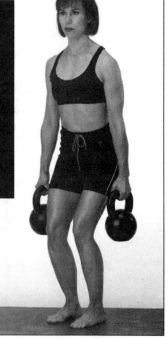

One-Arm Deadlift

A tip for stricter performance: You will have to keep your whole core very tight. Focus especially on your oblique and glute on the side opposite the kettlebell.

Finish standing straight and strong. Let some—but not all!—of your air out, inhale again, and descend following the standard box squat "groove." Let the weight of the kettlebell completely rest on the ground, and totally relax your body before tightening up for another rep.

You will be pleased with the firm, powerful feeling throughout your body. And the hip- and waist-toning effects of the one-arm deadlifts will start showing immediately.

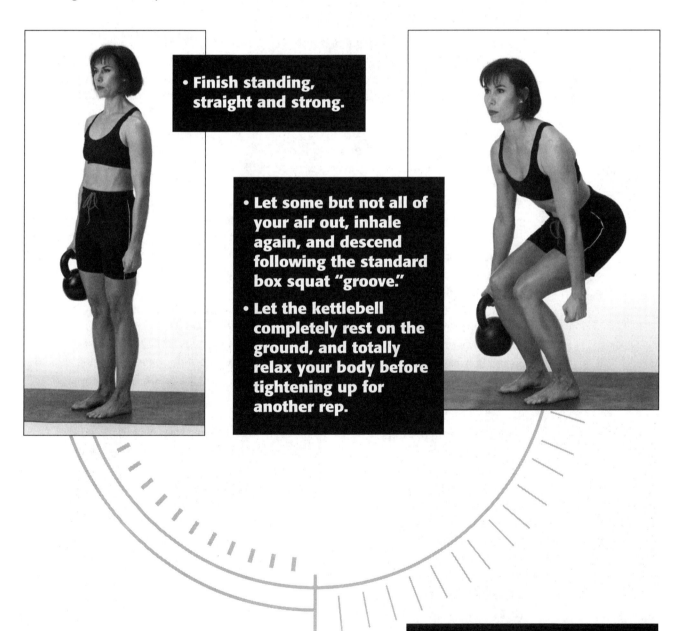

• Finish standing, straight and strong.

• Let some but not all of your air out, inhale again, and descend following the standard box squat "groove."

• Let the kettlebell completely rest on the ground, and totally relax your body before tightening up for another rep.

One-Arm Deadlift

Kettlebells deliver usable strength

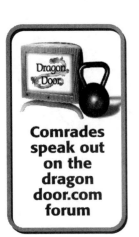

Comrades speak out on the dragon door.com forum

"She will stop a galloping horse and enter a burning house."
—Turgenev, Russian poet

Reaping the practical benefits of KB training: A testimonial
From: RCH

Moved to a new apartment this weekend. Did 4 hours of loading Friday after work; up at 6 a.m. Saturday for 2 1/2 hours of unloading. All by myself, mind you. Buddies all had better things to do, but I didn't mind. I was looking forward to it as a test. No ramp on the truck like last time; rather everything I owned got lifted and stacked. "Step-ups" into the truck over and over again.

The last time I moved by myself, I was beat up for days afterward. After a couple of months or so of KB training, I can say it has no doubt made a huge difference. I was barely sore when I woke up Sunday. I even did a light KB workout that morning!

Weird experience— maybe someone can explain
From: Vaughan

I did a particularly hard workout today with my KB, and my grip was extremely cooked—my forearm muscles burning. I picked up my Ivanko gripper, and I felt stronger with it then I ever had before. I closed it on a much higher setting.

Re: Cardio suggestions
From: David C.

The Russian Kettlebell Challenge is for you. The great thing about the workout is you not only gain cardio and endurance benefits, but you also get great functional strength benefits. The repeated practice of the basic movements of the snatch and clean-and-jerk greases the groove to unlocking your body's power. Basically, your entire body learns to be strong more efficiently and with less effort. (This is my understanding of the theory as well as my experience. It's easier to pick up and move furniture all day, carry fertilizer, etc.) This just might be the most efficient workout you can find.

KB magic
From: aet51

I went to Duluth this weekend to do some skiing. I nailed a jump going way too fast and started to do a back flip (an accident) and don't know what happened after that. Everyone who watched me wipe out thought I would be totally messed up, but all I ended up with were some strained muscles in my lower back and a real bad headache. I believe the KB's have turned me into a man of steel. I don't even think I'll be afraid to hit the same jump next time I go.

Re: Pavel, Jump experience!
From: tonya1980

Absolutely! My gear weighs nothing, and that goes for everything. Earlier this week, I qualified on the SAW and M-16, and those things weighed nothing. My shot group tightened up considerably, especially in the prone unsupported position. For the first time, I was able to literally shoot the middle out of the target when we did NBC fire. Heck, my Plt. Sgt. is seriously considering giving me a SAW for good and giving my M-16 to a SAW gunner.

Yes, my [parachute] landing did feel a lot more "together"—safer and softer.

Re: Re: Kettlebell convincing
From: Braveheart

I'm now using the KBs exclusively. I don't have the time to go to the gym with school, work, karate, and softball plus a personal life. They give me all I need, and that is functional strength and energy so I can perform better in all my activities. You will not be disappointed.

Firm and shrink your waist, boost your overall strength, and protect your back with the POWER BREATHING CRUNCH

*"The crunch belongs on the junk pile
of history next to communism."*

I have spoken out against the conventional crunch in my *Bullet-Proof Abs* book, in magazine articles, at the dragondoor.com discussion site, and at the Coffee Bean across the street. The conventional crunch does not work the abs effectively, hurts many Comrades' backs and necks, and plainly puts one in a state of hypnotic trance: "You are getting sleepy . . . You are turning communist . . ."

Yet Americans persist with their favorite pastime. It's like I've been trying to tell you to say no to baseball. OK, I know you're going to keep crunching, so the least I can do is tell you how to make your crunch work.

Let's fix the neck discomfort first. There are three ways the crunch aggravates your neck

The first is pulling on your head with your hands. Don't! Reach your straight arms toward your feet along your body. It helps if you bend your wrists back and imagine that you are pushing with the bases of your palms, the power spots straight below the little fingers that martial artists use for breaking bricks.

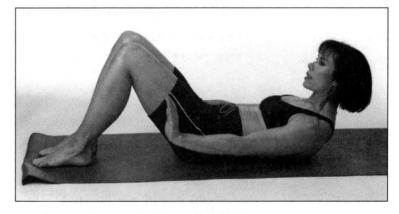

This suggested position is custom made for Comrades with bad necks because the act of reaching forward activates the muscles antagonistic to the traps. The latter get inhibited via the mechanism of reciprocal inhibition—in other words, your body has no desire to wear itself out by pressing the gas and the brake pedals at once.

Power Breathing Crunch

The second reason your neck gets aggravated by crunches is the fact that you are doing too many reps. Your melon weighs 15 pounds. Pump it up and down 20—or worse yet, 100 times—and you have got a problem. I have spoken out against high-rep ab training on many occasions, so I won't repeat myself. The

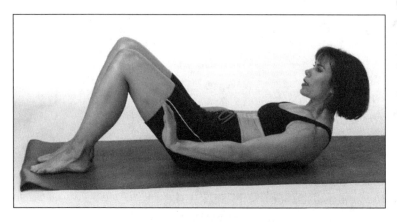

preferred set and rep scheme for your abs is 5x5, 2 to 7 times a week. Period. And if you want to build up a prominent six-pack, just double the number of sets but cut back your training frequency to 2 to 3 days a week. 'Nuff said.

Then there is the misplaced continuous tension, where the trainee keeps her neck off the floor and partially flexed for the duration of the set. To avoid the unnecessary neck strain and the shortening of the muscles in front of the neck that give you a chicken-like posture, lower your head under control all the way down to the floor and relax for a second before doing the next rep.

Once you've dealt with these three problems, you will most likely say good-bye to ab training–related neck problems once and for all.

- **Don't pull on your head with your hands!**
- **Reach your straight arms toward your feet along your body.**
- **Bend your wrists back and imagine that you are pushing a heavy object toward your feet with the bases of your palms.**
- **Reduce your volume of crunches to no more than 25 per workout in sets of no more then 5 reps, 2 to 7 times a week.**
- **Lower your head all the way down to the floor under control, and relax for a second before doing the next rep.**

The traditional crunch is a very subtle movement that simply fails to overload the abs of everyone but those few gifted individuals who have an unusually fine mind-muscle link. You will be able to dramatically increase the intensity of the abdominal contraction—and powerfully engage the rest of the muscles of your midsection—if you Power Breathe while crunching. Make sure to clear this technique with your doctor if you have a heart condition, hypertension, or other health concerns.

Power Breathing Crunch

Start by learning to breathe into your stomach. Here's one simple way: Lie down on the floor on your back. Place one shoe or book on your stomach and another on your chest. Now practice breathing until only the object on your belly moves up and down and the one on your chest stays put. Remember how it feels to breathe like this.

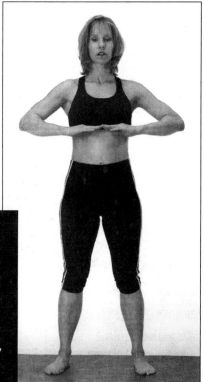

Now get up and practice the following martial arts drills before coming back for more crunches. Hold your hands at your sternum level. Keep your "energy" in your belly, not in your chest.

Take a diaphragmatic or belly breath, about three-quarters of the maximum volume of air your lungs can handle. At the same time, contract the muscles of the pelvic diaphragm as if you're trying to stop yourself from going to the bathroom. (Martial artists know how this odd technique increases power and promotes health.) Keep this anal lock while you exert yourself during each rep. This applies to all bodybuilding exertions, not just crunches. Relax the pelvic floor muscles between each rep.

- **Take a diaphragmatic breath, about three-quarters of your max.**
- **At the same time, pull up your pelvic floor.**
- **Keep your pelvic floor muscles tight during exertions; relax in between them.**

Press your tongue hard behind your teeth, and expel all your air under high pressure. Understand that just exhaling won't cut it. You must hiss like the air hose at a gas station that's used for filling tires—not like a leaking tire! To maximize the internal pressure, make sure to plug up your teeth with your tongue as tight as possible. And concentrate on squeezing all your waist muscles.

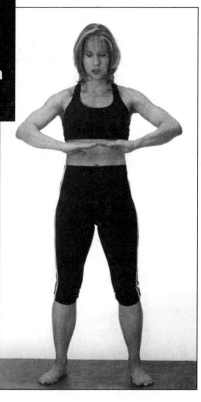

This doesn't mean sucking in your stomach! The misguided advice to pull your belly button toward your spine severely compromises the effectiveness of your abdominal training. First, the abdominal wall gets concave, and your muscles are supposed to contract in a straight line, not an arc. Second, contrary to popular belief, this maneuver fails to engage the belt-like transversus abdominis that wraps your waist beneath your abs and compresses your viscera. An experiment with the so-called vacuum drill will illustrate this point. Expel all your air, and then expand your ribcage to the max without inhaling. Your stomach will suck in as your diaphragm pulls up like a plunger into the low-pressure zone above.

Power Breathing Crunch

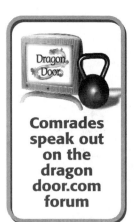

Shrink your waist with Power Breathing

Lost an inch off my waist due to tension techniques :-)

From: DaveBrown

I attended Pavel's AWESOME class in Denver last weekend and have had a great side-effect. The class concentrated a lot on tension techniques. From using these techniques for my abs during lifting and consciously thinking to keep them tense all day (no sagging allowed, makes my back hurt), my abs are now tighter and my waist is smaller.

On the other hand, just focusing on compressing the air in your stomach will recruit your transversus abdominis and compact your waist naturally at the end of the exhalation. Save up some dough to buy the pair of smaller pants that you might need a few weeks later. Power Breathing will shrink your waist by tightening up your transversus abdominis.

Don't send the pressure into your chest or head. Although you might get slightly light headed, you shouldn't feel the pressure upstairs! Direct the Power Breath into your stomach. Literally push down with your hands, as shown in the photo, and imagine that a plunger is coming down and dividing your lungs and your stomach. The 'plunger' is your diaphragm, a parachute shaped muscle, at work. Don't make faces either—just keep a tight tongue.

Completely relax once you have gotten rid of your air. Chill for as long as you want until the next rep so you don't get dizzy.

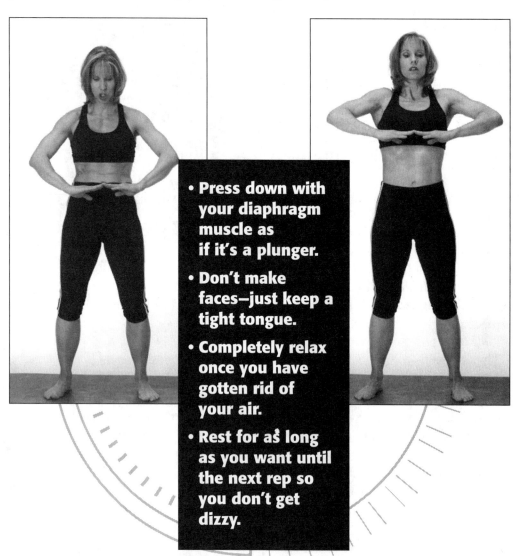

- Press down with your diaphragm muscle as if it's a plunger.

- Don't make faces—just keep a tight tongue.

- Completely relax once you have gotten rid of your air.

- Rest for as long as you want until the next rep so you don't get dizzy.

Power Breathing Crunch

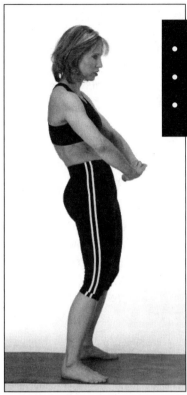

- **Round your spine.**
- **Tense your glutes.**
- **"Tuck in your tail."**

Now that you've done 2 or 3 Power Breaths, let's make them even more effective. Make a point of rounding your spine, tensing your glutes, and "tucking in your tail." Feel those dear abbies? It's amazing how much difference such subtle changes can make, isn't it?

Practice doing 5 to 10 Power Breaths a day for the first week of your _From Russia with Tough Love_ training. And a week later, you will be ready to hit the deck and take on the Power Breathing crunch.

Excel at sports with kettlebells

Re: Kettlebell testimonies
From: tylerhasselhoff
On the tennis court, I am much quicker and more explosive. My speed is now a weapon for me because I can get to just about any ball. My opponents have to play better as a result. I also have increased my endurance, both in short-term bursts, such as a tough point, and in the long-term, such as a long match. Kettlebells and Pavel's other programs are the only fitness programs that have ever given me results that translated into better play.

KB success story
From: blademaster
You know 'em, you love 'em, now it's time for another KB success story. I've used my KB for 4 workouts, and was playing baseball today. Got a hit, and I ran around the bases 2x faster than usual! Can't wait to see how I'm doing after a few months!

Re: KB success story
From: hanuman
I have noticed this also. I don't run for fitness or anything but when I have to run after my nephews... I seem a lot quicker and light on my feet. Isn't this called the "What the hell effect"? ...The guy I train with hasn't run in two months but placed fairly well in a local run in Philly. He trained only with KB before the event.

On KBs and water sports
From: warnerkallus
We began the water polo season last week, and after a summer without getting in the pool, I am a much stronger player. My recovery time is much less, and for a noodle arm, my shot has moved from "a firm pass" to actually demanding a little respect. In swimming, the cross-training effect is less except that I can hold higher levels of effort longer.

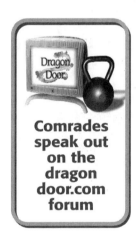

Comrades speak out on the dragon door.com forum

Power Breathing Crunch

Excel at sports with kettlebells (continued)

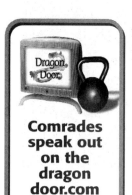

Comrades speak out on the dragon door.com forum

Kettlebell carryover to volleyball = success
From: majorwoody

I want to relate to the Party my success in the brief time I've been slinging around my puny 1-pood kettlebell, more specifically as it relates to recovery. For over a month, my volleyball team hasn't played in a tournament due to scheduling conflicts, injuries, etc., and during that time, I've been practicing mostly the ballistic drills, swings, and one-armed snatches with some military presses thrown in. Well, after an all-day tournament yesterday, with 6 matches that lasted up to an hour each, I finally got to see what everyone has been raving about for myself. Although I didn't notice an increase in my vertical leap, I was able to jump just as high and come in for my approaches just as fast at the very end of the day as at the beginning. I play one of the most physically demanding positions in volleyball, middle blocker, and normally the day after a tournament, I can hardly walk and experience delayed-onset muscle soreness in nearly every muscle in my body, especially my abs and legs. But I woke up this morning with hardly any ill effect. It's unbelievable! I'm the grizzled veteran on my team at 34, but after long rallies, when my much younger teammates were sucking wind, I felt fine. And after the last match, when they were all hobbling around, moaning and groaning, I felt fresh as a daisy. Who knew kettlebells could have such a profound effect?

Re: Alpine skiing
From: little bear

Kettlebells, hands down. These hunks of iron seem to be custom made for alpine skiing. Core strength is as important, or more so, than leg strength in skiing. With RKC', you will kick the crap out of moguls and everything else will seem like a walk in the park. Interestingly, after RKC' with only dumbbells last year, I had absolutely none of the beginning-of-season stiffness. By the way, I ski 100+ days per year, competed at the national level in my youth, as well as coached up until just recently.

KBs and swimming
From: sok

I'm a lousy swimmer. I've been doing KBs for about 2 months now, and last week, I got a pool membership so I can pass the Marine Corps swim test. I can definitely feel that the KB has helped my strokes—important things like breath control and relaxation. I'll just have to learn by "getting wet," but the KB has definitely helped me in my swimming.

Re: Kettlebells meet Aikido
From: Aiki4me

As you can tell by my nick, Aikido is my chosen martial art. I have had the same observations. I have been training RKC' since October—first with the 1 pood and added the 1.5 about 2 months ago. I often get to be the crash test dummie (uke) for tests. During and after Randori, I would be sweating buckets and sucking wind. Now I barely break a sweat and don't get winded hardly at all. Not bad for a 45-year-old smoker—soon to be ex-smoker. A few more things I noticed:
1. Better connection with Nage's center.
2. Shock resistance improved.
3. Wrist strength improved greatly. (Handy when working with newbies on Nikyo and Kotegashi.)
4 Improvement in Ki extension.
5. Hand and foot speed is faster.
6. Two-year-old shoulder injury is much better than before. (Injured when my arm collapsed during a standing forward roll.)

Re: Kettlebell testimonies (bit long)
From: WillToPower

I shaved 2 minutes off my run time in the mile and a half portion of the PFT for the state police in just 2 weeks.

Lie on your back, your feet flat and your knees at a 45 degree angle. Place your arms along your body, as described earlier. Now slowly crunch up as you Power Breathe. Pause at the top of the movement long enough to expel the last bit of air. You will experience a tremendous contraction—and have the abs to show for it.

Come down and relax. Rest your head on the floor between repetitions. You may inhale on the way down or wait until you hit the deck, your choice. Focus on the tension, not the reps.

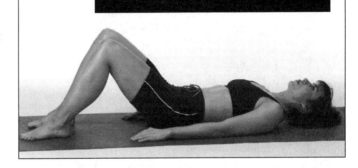

- **Relax your head on the floor between repetitions.**
- **Inhale on the way down or wait until you hit the deck, your choice.**
- **Focus on the tension, not the reps.**

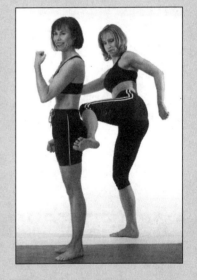

Body hardening for teaching tightness

Do you have a hard time tensing up a muscle group? Then teach yourself how with the practice of controlled striking. I use this technique extensively with my military and law enforcement clients. The Marine Corps Martial Arts Program refers to controlled striking of your muscles as *body hardening*. For instance, if you have a hard time tucking your butt under during your crunches, a few friendly, firm but careful—kicks in the butt (not the tailbone!) will show you the way. Ditto for the glute tension needed for the standing version of Power Breathing.

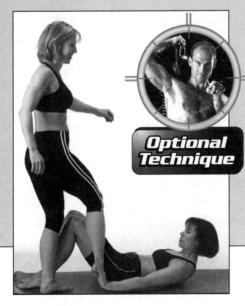

Optional Technique

Power Breathing Crunch

Protect your back with a virtual belt

It's estimated that a person leaning forward with a 175-pound weight will load his or her spine with over 2,200 pounds, which is a lot more than the spine can withstand. Yet powerlifters routinely lift a lot more than 175 pounds and even live to tell about it. Teenager Jennifer Maile just pulled a 403-pound women's open world record deadlift at a bodyweight of only 105 pounds!

Professor Vladimir Zatsiorsky explains that these estimates don't jibe with reality because they don't take into account intra-abdominal pressure, or IAP. "IAP increases during muscular efforts, especially during a Valsalva maneuver," writes Zatsiorsky. "As a result of internal support, the pressure on the intervertebral disks can be reduced by up to 20% on average and up to 40% in extreme cases."

When your spine is compressed by lifting heavy poundage, you cannot afford to lose any air, for it protects your back like an air cushion. So instead of forcefully expelling your breath, just *pretend* that you are. This is a technique I call Virtual Power Breathing.

Practice a couple of regular Power Breaths, as described earlier. Then do the same—but catch your breath in your throat instead of letting it escape. You will experience a comfortable tightness in your waist as your abdomen gets pressurized. Your belly should not stick out or suck in; it will just get rock hard, and you will feel very solid inside. Send the pressure to your belly, not your chest or your head! And make sure not to flex your spine. Try to maintain its normal curve.

If you don't have the kinds of medical restrictions discussed earlier, apply this virtual technique to any slow exertion that stresses out your spine: various deadlifts, squats, overhead presses, and so on. Better yet, use this technique when you are hauling heavy stuff outside the gym.

The effects of Virtual Power Breathing are nothing short of miraculous. The usually heavy weight will feel whimsically light, and your back won't likely feel anything at all.

- **Squeeze something between your knees during your ab work to emphasize the lower abs.**

Week 3 will have you blast the area that people incorrectly refer to as the lower abs, which is really the transversus abdominis and the muscles of the pelvic diaphragm. Sit on the floor with your hands on your knees. Flex your abs as hard as you can for a couple of seconds. Note the intensity of the contraction. Now slip your tennis shoes, pressed together sole to sole, between your knees and repeat the test—this time, trying to crush your shoes to pulp with your knees. I want to see gel squirting! You will be stunned at the tension generated in your lower abs! To emphasize this problem area, do your Power Breathing crunches while crushing the shoes or a ball between your knees.

Power Breathing Crunch

Learn a better contraction with a partner

You will get better at contracting your abs and other torso muscles if you practice your crunches with a partner a couple of times. Your partner should give you moderate resistance with her hands—not too easy yet not impossible to overcome. Both of you should make sure to position your hands in the CPR position, which doesn't tweak your wrists. Press with the bases of your palms.

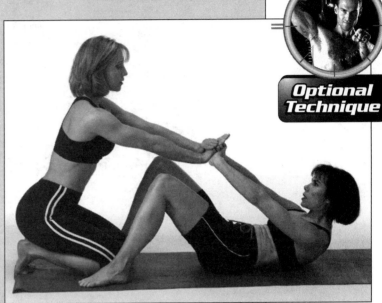

Optional Technique

You should notice a greater contraction of your abdominals. At the same time, your shoulders should perform an antishrug and your pecs and the other muscles connecting your arms to your torso should flex hard, as well. Remember this feeling for next time, when you do the drill by yourself.

During Week 4, the last week of Basic Training, you'll give your obliques something extra to worry about. Place your palms one atop the other, as if you are getting ready to give CPR, your elbows still straight. (By the way, you may use this position for the standard forward or knee squeeze crunches, as well.)

Instead if reaching straight ahead, push in the direction slightly outside one of your knees. Don't try to twist; just reach toward your knee. You may do all your reps on one side before switching to the other or alternate; it's up to you. Make a point of contracting the glute on the side you are pushing to the limit; it should feel like a hard wheel.

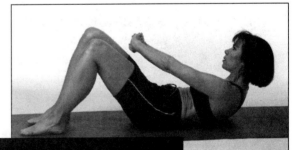

• Cramp the glute on the side you are pushing to; it should feel like a hard wheel.

Power Breathing Crunch

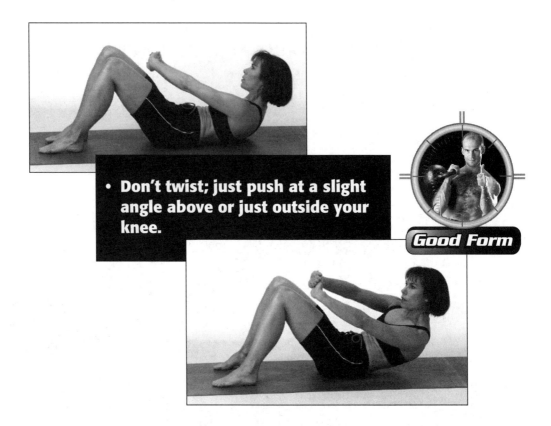

• Don't twist; just push at a slight angle above or just outside your knee.

Good Form

Get better results in fewer reps with a hot new technique

D. C.'s husband, Philadelphia's RKC-certified instructor Steve Maxwell, M.S., developed a unique high-tension technique of *forced rep reduction*. Instead of encouraging his clients at Maxercise to try harder and do more reps, Steve tells them to try harder and do less!

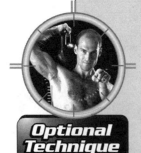

Optional Technique

Before you get indignant at this apparent violation of the progressive overload dogma, flex your brain a little. The harder you squeeze your glutes, the more you will inhibit the hip flexors and the harder your abs will work. And the fewer reps, you will manage. The harder you pressurize your abdomen with Power Breathing, the more resistance the air and your viscera will provide. And so the rep count drops even further while your abs, obliques, and internal muscles get the workout of a lifetime.

Now that I am done digitally remastering this ineffective oldie, about the only thing that's left of the traditional crunch is the name. So much the better. It's time you got results for a change.

Power Breathing Crunch

From Russia with Tough Love
Advanced Training: Weeks 5-8

1 **Deck or low box squat—4x RM**
     Alternated with the two-arm swing—4x10
     Knee-squeeze Power Breathing crunch—4x4
     Assisted clean—4x4 per arm

2 **Two-arm swing—2x10**
     Alternated with the "Good Morning" stretch—2x5
     Angled Power Breathing crunch—2x2 per side
     Assisted clean—2x4 per arm

3 **Deck or low box squat—3xRM**
     Alternated with the two-arm swing—3x20
     Knee-squeeze Power Breathing crunch—4x4
     Clean—4x4 per arm

4 **Deck or low box squat—1x1/2 RM**
     "Good Morning" stretch—2x5
     Angled Power Breathing crunch—2x2 per side
     Assisted clean—2x4 per arm

5 **Deck or low box squat—2xRM**
     Alternated with the two-arm swing—2x30
     Knee-squeeze Power Breathing crunch—4x4
     Clean—2x8 per arm

6 **Two-arm swing—1x20**
     "Good Morning" stretch—2x5
     Angled Power Breathing crunch—2x2 per side
     Assisted clean—2x8 per arm

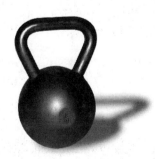

7 **Relax!**

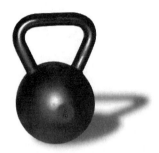

Kettlebells raise hell at a health club

The kettlebell dialogues
From: Rob Lawrence

Since a couple of Comrades have wondered aloud, "What happens when you take a kettlebell into a commercial gym?" I'd like to present the following dialogues, all real-life examples from my own experience.

Very Big Guy (Brooklynite): "Hey, wat is dat?"
RL: "It's called a 'kettlebell.' It's Russian."
VBG: (Picks it up.) "Hey, it's heavy."
RL: "This is a one-arm snatch." (Demonstrates snatch.)
VBG: "Cool."
One week later.
VBG: (On seeing RL) "Hey, where's the ball thing?"
RL: (Leaves room to get drink of water)

Slouchy-looking liberal bearded type: (Attempts to pick up and move kettlebell. Drops it.) "Hey, what the hell is that?"
RL: (Returns, glares. Picks up kettlebell.)
SLLBT: (Says nothing. Moves quietly to other side of room.)

Girl: "Hey, that thing looks like Mickey Mouse."
RL: "It's called a 'kettlebell.'"
Girl: "It looks like Mickey Mouse."
RL: (Silence.)

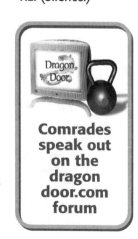

Comrades speak out on the dragon door.com forum

Keep lowering the squat box depth, if you're ready for it.

1 **One-legged deadlift—5x4 per leg**
Assisted military press—4x3
Box front squat—3x5 per side
One-arm swing—2x20 per arm

2 **Power Breathing crunch—4x5**
Clean—1x10 per arm
Assisted military press—2x3

3 **One-legged deadlift—4x5 per leg**
Military press—4x2
Box front squat—4x5 per side
One-arm swing—2x25 per arm

4 **Power Breathing crunch—3x5**
Assisted clean—1x10 per arm
Assisted military press—2x4

5 **One-legged deadlift—5x5 per leg**
Military press—4x3
Box front squat—5x5 per side
One-arm swing—2x30 per arm

6 **Power Breathing crunch—2x5**
Assisted clean—1x10 per arm
Assisted military press—2x4

7 **Relax!**

ADVANCED TRAINING: WEEK 7

If you can't do free front and overhead squats, use the box.

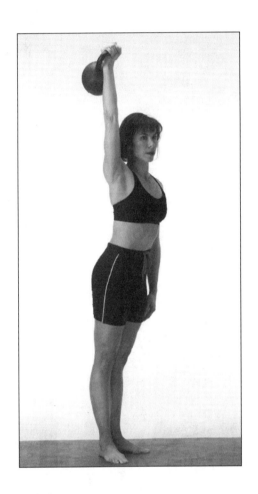

1   **Military press—4x3**
    Overhead squat—3x2
    Front squat—2x5 per side
    One-arm swing—2x20 per arm

2   **Clean and military press—3x3 (drop and reclean the KB after each rep)**
    Turkish getup—5x1 per arm
    Rolling situp—2x2 circles in each direction

3   **Military press—4x4**
    Overhead squat—3x2
    Front squat—3x5 per side
    One-arm swing—4x15 per arm

4   **Clean and military press—3x3**
    Turkish getup—6x1 per arm
    Rolling situp—2x2 circles in each direction

5   **Military press—4x5**
    Overhead squat—3x3
    Front squat -3x5 per side
    One-arm swing—3x20 per arm

6   **Clean and military press—3x3**
    Turkish getup—7x1 per arm
    Rolling situp—2x2 circles in each direction

7   **Relax!**

ADVANCED TRAINING: WEEK 8

Don't progress to more challenging windmills unless you feel ready. Also make sure to terminate the sets of the combination exercise before your form slips in any of the component drills. **(Exercises next page)**

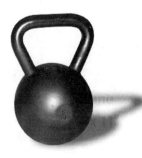

ADVANCED TRAINING: WEEK 8

1 Military press—3x3
"Good Morning" stretch—2x5
Windmill with kettlebell below—3x3 per side
One-arm swing—1x10 per arm
Clean—1x10 per arm
Snatch—1x10 per arm
Two-arm swing—1x RM

2 Knee-squeeze Power Breathing crunch—3x5
Bottoms-up clean—4x3 per arm
Overhead squat—2x5 per side

3 Military press—3x3
"Good Morning" stretch—2x5
Windmill with kettlebell below—3x3 per side
Windmill with kettlebell above—2x2 per side
One-arm swing—1x10 per arm
Clean-and-press—1x10 per arm
Snatch—2x10 per arm
Front SQ—1x RM on weaker side, then same number of reps on stronger side

4 Knee-squeeze Power Breathing crunch—3x5
Bottoms-up clean—2x2 per arm
Bottoms-up clean-and-press—3x1
"Good Morning" stretch—2x5

5 Windmill with kettlebell below—1x5 per side
Windmill with kettlebell above—2x2 per side
Windmill with two kettlebells—2x2 per side
Combination exercise (swing, clean-and-press, snatch, overhead squat) 3x RM per side
Deck squat—1x RM

6 "Good Morning" stretch—2x5
Windmill with hand behind back—2x4 per side
Knee-squeeze Power Breathing crunch—3x5
Bottoms-up clean—2x2 per arm
Bottoms-up clean-and-press—5x2 per arm

7 Relax!

Get super flexible and work your hips and thighs even harder with the DECK SQUAT

By now, you must have significantly increased your box squat depth. Your legs are firming up, and your newly found hip and knee mobility makes you feel like dancing. Some of you are ready to take the rocking squat one step deeper and harder by squatting to the floor.

Note that you will really have to punch that kettlebell forward and keep your momentum going if you are to get up (although at some point, you may get strong, light, and flexible enough to rock up slowly—an advanced dimension in pain).

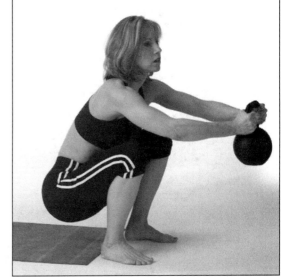

Simplify with kettlebells

Re: Re: No disrespect, but . . .
From: bulldog
Look at this way. Even if you purchased the video and a couple of kettlebells to get started, you can completely train your whole body (strength and endurance) for a fraction of the cost of a treadmill and weights. In addition, KBs don't take up any space and they will last forever. They are also great fun!
I don't care what you say as a conditioning tool—original bells are by far the best. Put them up against whatever you want. K-bells rule!

Just a thought
From: mlilley
No wonder KB's were the choice of exercise in Russia. In my basement gym, I have over 1000 pounds of free weights and bench, a treadmill, a stationary bike, and yes (go ahead, laugh at me), even a Bow Flex. But if I had to make a choice and only keep one item to stay in shape

(especially if the wife kicked me out—LOL), I'd take them trusty little nasty KB's. I've lifted since I was 14 and pushed it hard and made some good gains the last 2 years. But for practical, down-and-dirty get me into shape, you can't beat the KB.

Smart decision
From: ScotPower
The kettlebells seem expensive at first, but even two full sets are a drop in the bucket in the long run, especially given the amazingly effective (and time-efficient) workouts you can do.

Re: Going back to the gym
From: David C.
For the cost of 1 month's gym membership, you can buy a heavy dumbell (or two) to do KB workouts. For the price of 2 months' membership, you can buy a small KB. Unless you live in a closet or can't exercise outside, gym memberships aren't worth it. Simplify.

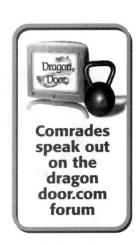

Comrades speak out on the dragon door.com forum

Deck Squat

Also, unless you are a yoga mutant, you won't be able to maintain an arched back in the rock-bottom position. Since you won't be holding a heavy barbell on your shoulders, this shouldn't be a problem unless you have a medical condition.

Otherwise, the technique is no different from the box squat. I told you: Once you get the basics down, learning the new *From Russia with Tough Love* stuff will be a breeze. That doesn't mean, though, that you should jump to deck squats before you have mastered low box squats. Slow and steady—that old thing.

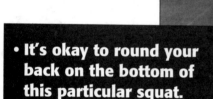

Good Form

- It's okay to round your back on the bottom of this particular squat.
- Punch the kettlebell far forward and keep your momentum going to get up.

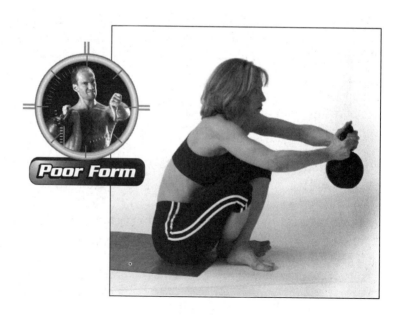

Poor Form

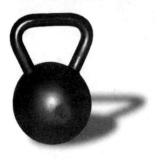

Deck Squat

Melt fat without the dishonor of doing aerobics and blast your hips and inner thighs with the SWING

David Willoughby, a weightlifting champion from the 1920s and an unquestionable authority on the iron game, stated that the two-arm swing "brings into action and develops practically every group of muscles on the back of the body and legs, and a good many others besides. . . . If you have time on your schedule for only one back exercise, make it this one."

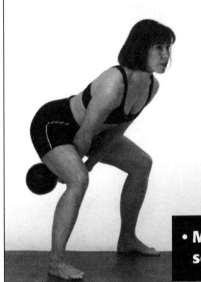

• **Maintain the squat alignment.**

Pick up a kettlebell with both hands, keeping your knees slightly bent, your back arched, your head up, and your weight on your heels. Swing the bell back between your legs. Observe how your weight remains on your heels and how your shins are vertical. No surprise! It looks just like the squat you have been doing.

Warning!

Kettlebell exercises can be dangerous. Don't hesitate to get rid of your kettlebell(s) if you are about to lose control or something goes wrong (for example, your shoulder is about to get wrenched). Just drop the kettlebell(s)! If your body is in the position where it might get hit by the falling weight, vigorously push the kettlebell(s) away from your body and let the kettlebell(s) fall.

A falling kettlebell(s) may damage property. If dropped on a hard surface, the kettlebell(s) may be damaged, too. To prevent either type of damage, it's strongly recommended that you practice on a soft surface outdoors.

Swing

You should feel that the K-bell is pulling you backward and loading your hamstrings. Snap the hips through by contracting your glutes explosively, a motion similar to a vertical jump. Visualize jumping up and at the same time projecting the KB straight ahead with the power of your hips. As with the squats, no lame scooping forward or bending over! This movement is a lot like the "bend-and-snap" that broke the UPS man's nose in the movie *Legally Blonde*.

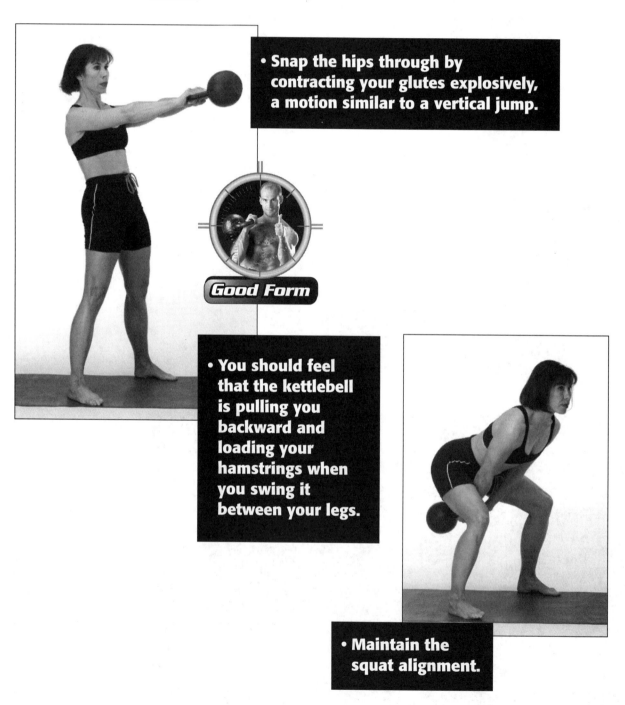

• **Snap the hips through by contracting your glutes explosively, a motion similar to a vertical jump.**

Good Form

• **You should feel that the kettlebell is pulling you backward and loading your hamstrings when you swing it between your legs.**

• **Maintain the squat alignment.**

Swing

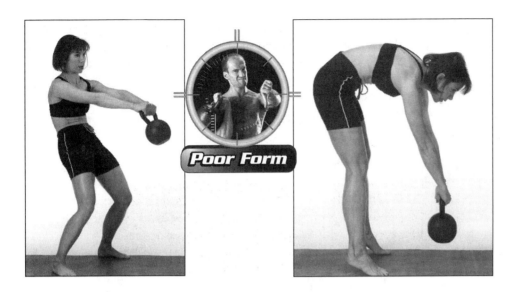

Poor Form

Get younger and healthier with kettlebells

Dr. Krayevskiy—the founder of the St. Petersburg Athletic Club, the father of Russian athletics, and the coach of "famous in the beginning of the XX century lifter and wrestler Russian Lion" Hackenschmidt—trained religiously with kettlebells. The doctor took up training at the age of 41, and 20 years later, he was said to look fresher and healthier than at 40.

Many Russians throw their KBs around noncompetitively, just for health. Vasiliy Kubanov, from a village in the Kirovograd area, underwent a very complex digestive tract surgery at 29 years of age. He was in such rough shape that the Soviet government (not famous for being too nice to anyone) offered to put him on disability. Vasiliy refused, started exercising with dumbbells and finally kettlebells, and even earned his national ranking in the sport of kettlebell lifting 4 years after his surgery!

A popular "Kettlebells for Health" movement was started by Evgeniy Revuka, who used to be the proverbial 98-pound weakling, plagued by various illnesses. Following some serious KB training, Revuka said good-bye to his sicknesses and became one of the top *gireviks* in the Ukraine. Inspired, he organized a kettlebell club at his factory, *Ukrelectorchermet*. The Comrades who joined boasted a long list of maladies—but not for long. Kettlebell training cured them.

Many Russians have successfully rehabilitated hopeless back injuries with kettlebells. Vladimir Nedashkovskiy, from the city of Uzhgorod, received a bad back injury back in 1969 but rehabbed himself with kettlebell lifting and even earned a national ranking! But the most inspiring story is that of Valentin Dikul. A circus acrobat, Dikul took a bad fall and broke his back when he was 17. He said no to a wheel chair and painstakingly rehabilitated himself, largely with the help of his trusted kettlebells. He did not stop there, either. He proceeded to become a great circus strongman, juggling 80-kilogram metal balls. Recently, at the age of 60, Dikul pulled a semiofficial all-time historic deadlift of 460 kilograms, or 1,015 pounds. (I say *semiofficial* because it was the Guinness people, rather than the International Powerlifting Federation, who certified it)!

If you have a back problem, make sure to check kettlebell or any other forms of exercise with your doctor before starting. No doubt, kettlebell lifting has a lot to offer toward improving your health, but it could also destroy you if you are not careful or take it up against your doctor's advice. Respect all power tools!

Swing

Repetitive ballistic loading of KB swings and snatches appears to be highly beneficial to your joints—provided you don't overdo it. Drs. Verkhoshansky and Siff state in *Supertraining* that "joints subjected to heavy impact are relatively free of osteoarthritis in old age and those subjected to much lower loading experience a greater incidence of osteoarthritis and cartilage fibrillation." After citing a long list of references, they continue:

> Dr. Mark Swanepoel, at the University of the Witwatersrand in South Africa, pointed out that, as one progresses up the lower extremity, from the ankle, to the knee, the hip and finally to the lumbar spine, so the extent of fibrillation increases at any given age. It appears that the cartilage of joints subjected to regular impulsive loading with relatively high contact stresses is mechanically much stiffer and better adapted to withstand the exceptional loading of running and jumping than the softer cartilage associated with low loading. Thus, joint cartilage subjected to regular repetitive loading remains healthy and copes very well with impulsive loads, whereas cartilage that is heavily loaded infrequently softens... The collagen network loses its cohesion and the cartilage deteriorates. (Swanepoel, 1998)

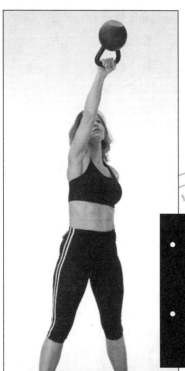

You may swing to different levels: your hips, your waist, or, as shown in the photo, your chest. The heavier the kettlebell, the lower you will be tempted to swing it—but that doesn't mean that you should not be doing low swings for high reps with a light bell. You may even swing higher but not so high that the bell will flip over your wrist. (That would be a snatch, and you don't know how to do one safely yet.)

- **Imagine shooting the kettlebell out through your straight arms at the chosen level.**
- **The kettlebell should align itself straight with your arms.**

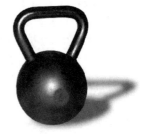

Swing

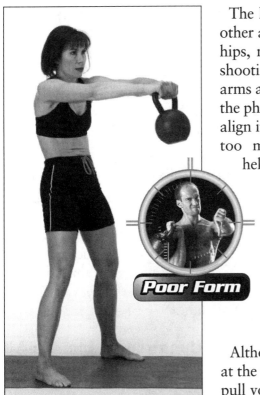

Poor Form

The key to the kettlebell swing, as to many other athletic endeavors, is to drive with your hips, not your arms and shoulders. Imagine shooting the KB out through your straight arms at the chosen level; look at the arrow on the photo. If you do it right, the kettlebell will align itself straight with your arms. If you use too much shoulder, the bell will dangle helplessly, as shown.

You'll find that your inner thighs and hamstrings will have to initiate the pull and your glutes will have to finish it. Cramp your glutes at the top of the movement. Lock your knees by firming your quads or pulling up your kneecaps.

Although your heels may come off the floor at the top of the swing, don't let the kettlebell pull you forward and overstress your back.

You'll find that your inner thighs and hamstrings will have to initiate the pull and your glutes will have to finish it. Cramp your glutes at the top of the movement. Lock your knees by firming your quads or pulling up your kneecaps.

Although your heels may come off the floor at the top of the swing, don't let the kettlebell pull you forward and overstress your back.

- **Cramp your glutes at the top of the movement.**
- **Lock your knees by firming your quads or pulling up your kneecaps.**
- **Although your heels may come off the floor at the top of the swing, don't let the kettlebell pull you forward and overstress your back.**

When you have reached the top of the movement, immediately let the KB freefall to the spot slightly below and behind your knees. Sit back and squat at the same time. Once you've reached the lowest point, explosively reverse the movement. Proceed with the next lift without hesitation. Don't pause at all. You have touched a hot stove!

Swing

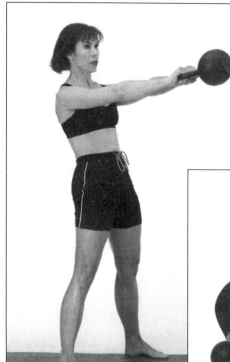

- **When you have reached the top of the movement, immediately let the bell freefall to the spot slightly below and behind your knees.**

- **Sit back and squat at the same time.**

- **Once the kettlebell is at the lowest point, explosively reverse the movement.**

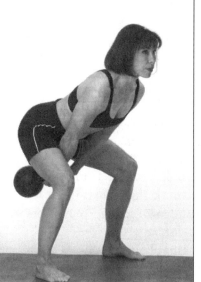

Synchronize your breathing with the movement. If you fail to find a rhythm, you won't be able to keep up for long. It helps to grunt on the top of the movement and pressurize your core. Your belly should feel the way it does when you are Power Breathing.

- **Synchronize your breathing with the movement.**

- **Grunt on the top of the movement and pressurize your core as if you are Power Breathing.**

A pleasant surprise

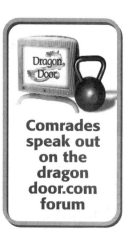

Comrades speak out on the dragon door.com forum

Swing

KB testimonial- unusual effects?
From: john44

I realize I'm preaching to the converted here, but I've found an interesting side effect(for me, anyway)in kb ballistics. For most of the past month, I have limited myself to ballistic drills at home, partially due to a minor stroke and its attendant side effects. Naturally I have been concerned about the effect of my lifting on blood pressure. Over several days, I have taken my BP before and after workouts, and after a particularly strenuous one got these results—before,170/109,after,145/88. My workout consisted of 2kb clean and jerks—10x6 total sets, along with 4 sets 1 arm snatch 10-8 reps each. All with 1 poods.

KB swings and abs
From: Paul Williams

I've been doing swings with my 1-and-a-bit-pood concrete KB, starting with 15 reps and adding 5 per week. I let the KB swing back as far as possible each time and start each swing by tensing my abdomen. My abs and adductors are getting quite a bit of work, which surprised me some, as I expected to feel it mainly along the back.

Re: KB swings and abs
From: Boicis EUR

I feel exactly the same, and that's also why I like it. I guess this drill requires balanced ab and back work.

KIAI! Your way to super strength

In any endeavor, mental focus delivers more than any physical transformation. Just watch a wiry old karate master chop a pile of bricks in half, a feat that would send a young bodybuilder to the emergency room. You can learn to focus your scattered strength through pressurized martial arts–style breathing.

Think of your brain as a CD player. Think of your muscles as speakers. Where do you think the amplifier is? In your stomach! Special *baroreceptors* measure the intra-abdominal pressure (IAP) and act as the volume control knob. When your IAP bottoms out, the tension in all your muscles drops off. In my book Relax into Stretch, I explain how to take advantage of this phenomenon and make dramatic gains in flexibility overnight.

On the other hand, when your internal pressure goes up, your nervous system gets more excited and the motoneurons, the nerve cells supplying your muscles, become more sensitive to the commands from your brain. So by cranking up the IAP volume knob, you automatically get noticeably stronger, in every muscle in your body and in any exercise!

I like demonstrating this concept in my seminars by having two students squeeze each other's hands as hard as possible. They rest for a minute and then repeat the test. One of the students does his old gig; the other is instructed to Power Breathe and "send energy from his stomach into his hand." The former student never fails to rub his or her hand in amazement.

Make sure that only one of the subjects engages in Power Breathing on the second trial, otherwise both will get stronger and not appreciate the gain. It's just like in the commercial where an employee asks his boss for a raise. The big shot counters, "Then I would have to give everyone else a raise as well, right? You would still be making less money than anyone else, so a raise really wouldn't solve anything, would it?"

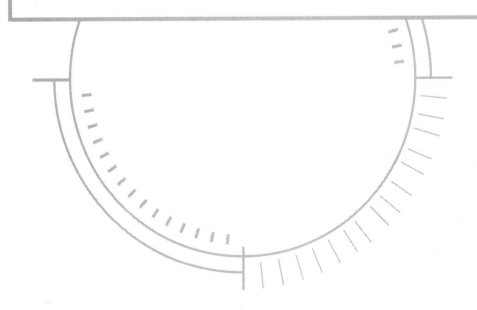

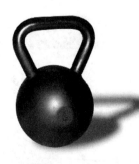

Swing

Once you have mastered the two-arm swing, you should try the one-arm version. You may pass the bell from hand to hand on the bottom or the top of the pull, if you have confidence in your timing and coordination.

Once you have finished a workout that involves swings or snatches, stretch your back and hamstrings. You will be glad you did. Stretching your inner thighs wouldn't hurt, either. OK, who am I kidding? You will hurt, but at least you will have a fighting chance of getting out of bed the morning after without help. In case you are wondering how your hip adductors could be involved in a pulling motion, you are about to find out the hard way.

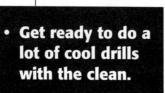

• **Get ready to do a lot of cool drills with the clean.**

Get ready to do a lot of cool drills with the CLEAN

The clean draws its name from the requirement to bring the weight to your shoulders in one clean movement. In the context of kettlebell training, it means swinging your KB between your legs until you hold the bell in the position shown. The clean can be used as an exercise or as a means to get the kettlebell to your shoulder safely for many other drills.

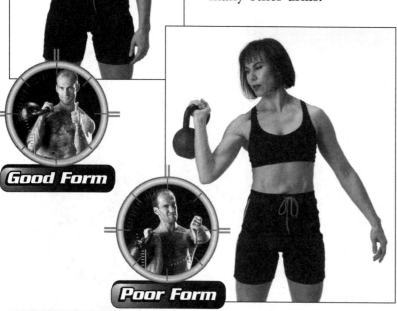

Good Form

Poor Form

Clean

Since many Comrades are tempted to unsafely backfist the kettlebell over the shoulder— which is bad news for the shoulder and elbow, as you might imagine—I strongly urge you to first practice with your free hand gripping over the hand holding the K-bell. Now, with your other arm restricting your movement, it would take a death wish to manage to fling the K-bell over your shoulder and away from your body.

The technique is identical for the one-arm clean and for the assisted clean. Pick up the kettlebell off the floor, and swing it back exactly the way you did for the swing drill. Keep your arm loose; the lifting is accomplished with your hip thrust. Keep your elbow in. Keep pulling. Quickly flip your elbow under when the bell has almost reached your shoulder. One more time: Do not pull with your arm! Although it may look like it in the photo, this is not an upright row!

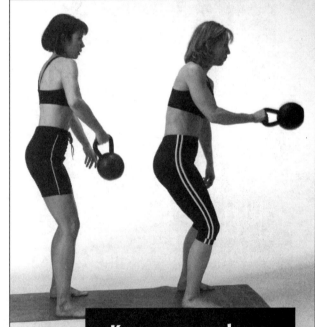

- To teach yourself to keep the kettlebell close to your body, start practicing with your free hand gripping over the hand holding the kettlebell.

- Swing your KB between your legs with the standard swing technique.

- Keep your arm loose, keep your elbow in, and quickly flip it under when the bell has almost reached your shoulder.

- This is not an upright row; the lifting is accomplished with your hip thrust.

Clean

Right before the hunk of iron has hit your forearm, quickly dip your knees and get under it. This action has been compared to putting on a sweater. Finish in the position shown.

Pay attention to proper wrist angle at the completion of the drill. Imagine that you are trying to wrap your fist in your forearm, toward the inside of your elbow. If you let you wrist hang free, as is your natural lazy tendency, you will be a hurting unit in no time flat.

• Squeeze the kettlebell's handle when its body is about to make contact with your forearm.

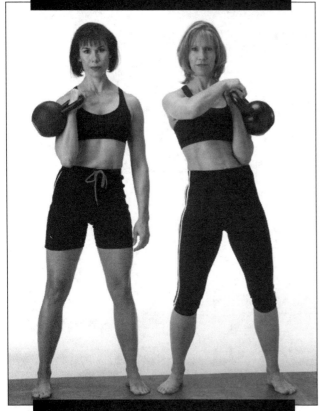

• Right before the kettlebell hits your forearm, quickly dip your knees and get under it.

• Treat your wrist as a rigid extension of your forearm; do not let it bend back.

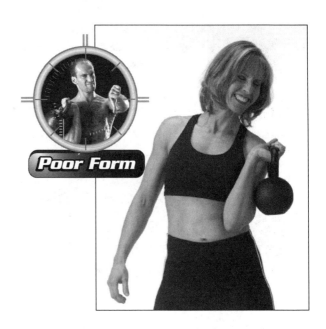

Poor Form

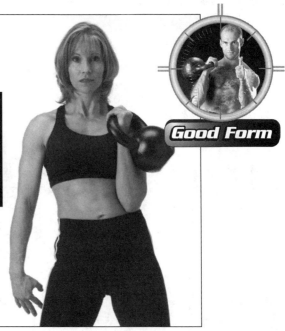

Good Form

Clean

The neutral wrist alignment applies to all the KB drills: cleans, snatches, presses, you name it. "The swinging of kettlebells requires a strong forearm and wrist," observed old-time strongman and wresting champion "Russian Lion" Hackenschmidt—and now you know that he wasn't kidding. Again, your wrist should be a rigid extension of your forearm. You will find that squeezing the bell's handle at the exact moment when the "cannon ball" is making contact with your forearm will make the bell land softer. Eventually, once you get the shock absorption technique down, you won't have to do it as much.

If you do the drill correctly, you will barely feel the impact of the bell on your forearm. It should be a kiss, not a punch. If you do not, you will get bruised or worse. Consider wearing a thick sweatshirt or something along those lines in the beginning—although Russians never do.

Kettlebells take so much control. Should I start on the machines?

Machine training is often hyped as the thing to do for beginners because free weights are harder to control. "Contrary to common belief," state Professor Verkhoshansky and Dr. Siff, *the novice must be taught from a base of mobility to progress to stability*, just as an infant learns to stand by first moving, staggering and exploring the environment." Would you like to be "staggering and exploring" while you are still relatively weak or later, when you have more strength to hurt yourself with?

The key to efficient and painless shock absorption is good technique. Every Independence Day, my wife Julie's family gathers at her Aunt Tootsie and Uncle John's cabin in the northern woods. The balloon toss is always a part of the holiday program. Couples get balloons filled with water and start passing them between one another. After every throw, everyone takes a step back. Sooner or later, the overfilled balloons get busted. Whoever keeps theirs alive the longest wins the jackpot. We always play with these at RKC instructor certification weekends and have a great time, especially if it's winter.

Shortly after you start playing this game, you realize that simply catching the blob is as good as throwing it against the wall. A sudden stop generates high Gs and bursts the bubble. You quickly learn to barely touch the balloon and rapidly retreat with it—to absorb the shock over a distance rather than at a dead stop.

Clean

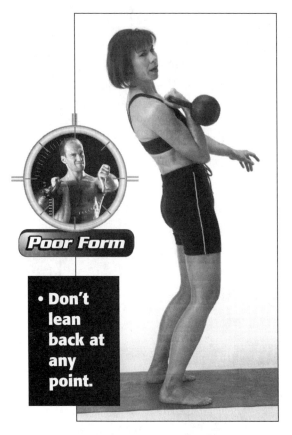

Poor Form

• Don't lean back at any point.

By the same token, the shock of the kettlebell coming down on your forearm should be absorbed by the long and smooth braking action of the knee dip, performed as the bell is flipping over the wrist and hitting the forearm. It's equally important to bring your elbow down as low as possible and to press your arm against your ribs. An arm that's "disconnected" from the body punishes the shoulder. Also imagine that the kettlebell is sort of like a glove you're putting on. As the bell/glove is moving in, the hand is moving in, too.

- **Absorb the shock of the kettlebell hitting your forearm over a distance through the smooth braking action of the knee dip.**

- **Bring your elbow down as low as possible, and press**

Don't lean back at any point! This applies to all the KB drills! And always brace your abs and glutes on impact!

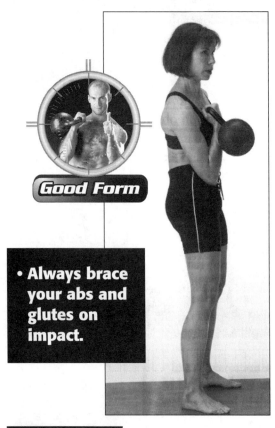

Good Form

• Always brace your abs and glutes on impact.

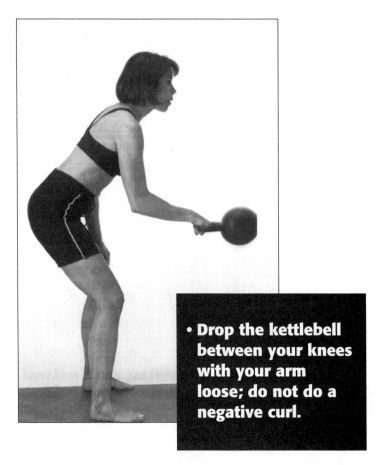

• Drop the kettlebell between your knees with your arm loose; do not do a negative curl.

Clean

Drop the kettlebell between your knees with your arm loose. Don't do a negative curl! You should absorb the shock with your hams—not your back or elbow!—as you have in doing swings. You may also find that squeezing the handle quickly at the lowest point will help to protect your elbows.

Then immediately reverse the movement. Be explosive!

No forearm bruising, please! Practice your cleans for very few sets and reps until you have gotten the "groove." And give your technique complete attention so it flows and doesn't hurt you. Two-handed practice will definitely help.

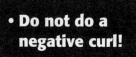

Poor Form

• Do not do a negative curl!

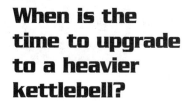

Good Form

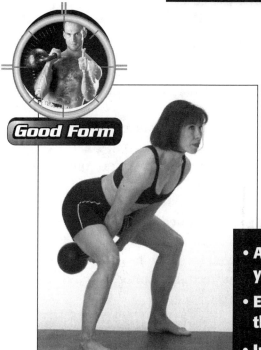

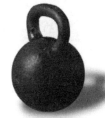

When is the time to upgrade to a heavier kettlebell?

I can't give you a better answer than "When it feels right." Heavier bells will deliver greater gains in strength and muscle tone. But don't discard your light ones, either; they will serve you well for an extra cardio kick and as a break on light days. A great schedule is to alternate between heavier and lighter bells from workout to workout.

• At the bottom position, absorb the shock with your hamstrings—not your back or elbow.

• Experiment with squeezing the handle quickly at the lowest point to unload the elbow.

• Immediately reverse the movement. Be explosive!

Clean

Add power and definition to your hips, thighs, and even abs with the FRONT SQUAT

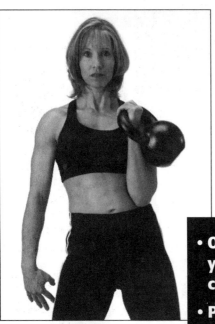

Anyone who has taken a yoga class knows that greater resistance doesn't necessarily mean you're working with a greater weight; it can mean you have poor leverage or a challenging load distribution. Squatting with the same kettlebell but held in the crook of your elbow—right where you have cleaned it—rather than in front of you, will suddenly make the squat more challenging. Let the kettlebell rest in the crook of your elbow—push your elbow forward and in. Besides, the K-bell is held on one side of your body, which will load one of your legs even more.

- **Once you have successfully cleaned your kettlebell, let it rest in the crook of your elbow.**
- **Push your elbow forward and in.**

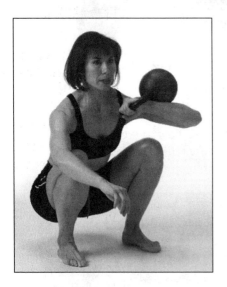

You will discover that the more arched and upright position dictated by the front squat delivers a real punch to your glutes and thighs. To make yourself even more miserable, once you have the flexibility and strength, try full front squats without a box.

Start by finding a comfortable squatting stance. Don't try to emulate the squatting stance of some woman who's in great shape. Her build, strength, and flexibility are different from yours, and copying her groove will do you no good.

Here's how to find a squatting stance suited to your body: Squat down on your haunches or as deep as you can. Shuffle your feet in and out, and play with the angle your feet are facing out. Persist until you find a position where your feet are planted flat and solid and your knees are tracking your feet.

You should be comfortable enough in this position to be able stay in it for a couple of minutes without propping yourself with your arms against your knees. It goes without saying that your knees should not bow in or protrude beyond your knees. (But I'll say it anyway.)

Front Squat

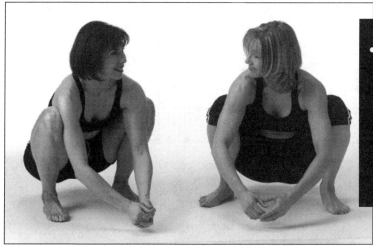

• You should be comfortable enough in this position to be able stay in it for a couple of minutes.

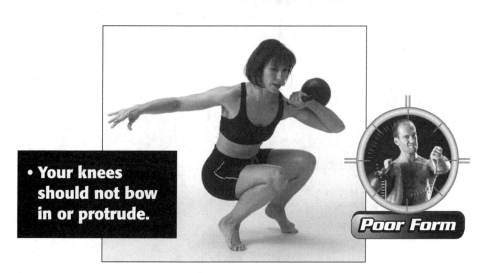

• Your knees should not bow in or protrude.

Poor Form

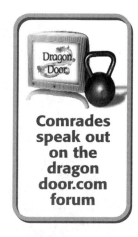

Comrades speak out on the dragon door.com forum

The Magic of K-bells of Different Weights

Re: Johnny pullups— 2 KB clean-and-press From: Rob Lawrence
The miracle of KBs, though, is that if you just keep hammering away, the totals go up. The work I do with the 36-pounders transfers to the 53's, which in turn transfers to the 72's. Beatific. Sometimes I think those KBs have halos—or wait, is it horns?

When you first tackle the box-free front squat, you probably won't be able to go rock bottom in good form. Either your knees will slip way forward and you won't be able to go any lower, or your back will round and your butt will tuck in. Unless you are exceptionally tight, you should be able to overcome this by contracting your hip flexors.

Here's how it is done: Stand on one foot with your knee up in the air. Push down on your knee with your hands, and feel the muscles on top of your thigh tense up. Remember that feeling and try to reproduce it when you are descending into a squat. Literally pull yourself down with your hip flexors. You will instantly notice that you can hit a greater depth with better form and control.

Take a belly breath before going down. Then descend, keeping a tight arch in your lower back. Once you have reached rock bottom, pressurize your abdomen using Virtual Power Breathing and straighten out. Push steadily, and don't let your butt shoot up before your shoulders.

Front Squat

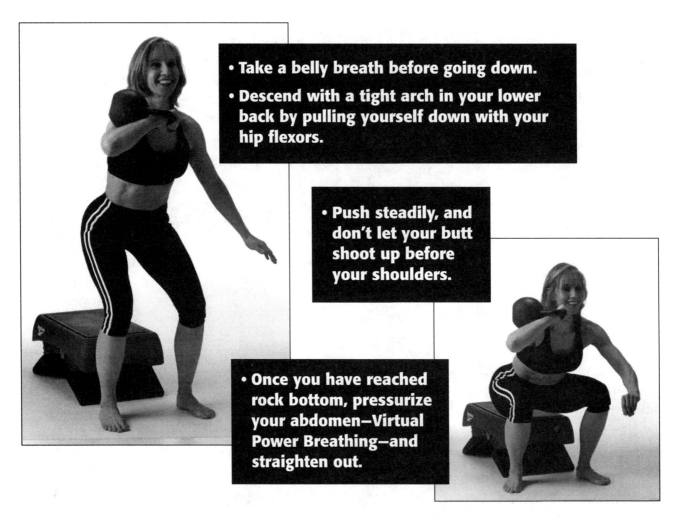

- **Take a belly breath before going down.**
- **Descend with a tight arch in your lower back by pulling yourself down with your hip flexors.**

- **Push steadily, and don't let your butt shoot up before your shoulders.**

- **Once you have reached rock bottom, pressurize your abdomen—Virtual Power Breathing—and straighten out.**

The countdown to shorts has started! Hot wheels, here you come!

Squat deeper and safer

Comrades speak out on the dragon door.com forum

Front Squat

Re: Full squats better than parallel?
From: Rob Lawrence

Over the past couple of weeks, I have begun a vigorous program of KB front squats—butt-to-heels as they say. I can honestly say that nothing has ever given me such an instant feeling of improved athleticism. I feel looser in the hips and can kick higher than I ever did while studying karate. As for running, it feels like someone finally took off the parking brake. If you can already front or back squat to the ground, I recommend that you go on doing so, particularly if it causes no knee problems. I favor the KB front squat because I feel it helps me go lower, while keeping my shins more or less vertical.

Abdominal pressure and squat depth
From: Rob Lawrence

Has anyone else noticed that there is a near-direct relationship between abdominal pressure and squat depth? If your body feels like the midsection is tight and under control, the lower extremities will relax and let you go deeper. But if your body senses any abdominal looseness, they will tighten and stop you in your tracks. Try experimenting with this.

Strengthen and firm your arms and shoulders with the MILITARY PRESS

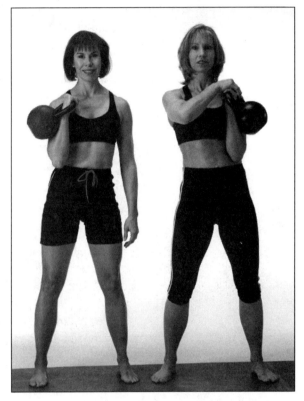

Women are smarter than men in emphasizing the lower body—the "rear-wheel drive," as RKC-certified instructor Tom Furman puts it—over the upper body. Athletically and functionally, it makes a lot more sense. *From Russia with Tough Love* accepts this enlightened attitude and focuses on your thighs, hips, and waist. Rest assured, though, that your arms and shoulder girdle won't be ignored. Enter the kettlebell military press, a totally different type of animal, if you compare it to your usual pressing exercises.

To start, clean the bell to your shoulder. You may clean-and-press the bell with both hands, if it's a little too heavy to manage one-handed. Maximally tighten your body on impact. It's not just about shock absorption; bracing for the weight will make the kettlebell feel like a toy in your hand, and your muscles will be powerfully loaded for action.

Anti-isolation for power and safety

One of the top reasons Comrades get injured in the gym is that they entertain the idiotic notion of isolation. Put it to rest! Isolation is neither possible nor desirable.

Make a fist—a white-knuckle fist! Observe how the tension involuntarily overflows from your forearm into your biceps, shoulder, even your pec. This is the neat "muscle software" called irradiation at work (See my book *Power to the People!: Russian Strength Training Secrets for Every American* for a detailed explanation.)

Counterintuitively, contracting muscles other than the ones directly responsible for the task at hand—the deltoids and triceps, in the case of the military press—does not take away from the power of the prime movers but instead amplifies it! This is especially true if it's the abs, the glutes, and the gripping muscles that you're flexing.

Military Press

In case you think that getting more "juice" into your arms by clenching your cheeks is preposterous, try this party trick: Give your friend the hardest handshake you can muster. (For obvious reasons, the guinea pig had better have a sturdy hand that can take it. Removing jewelry is also a good idea.) Shake off the tension, rest for a minute, and then repeat the test. This time, in addition to trying to demolish your Comrade's paw, flex your glutes as if you are trying to pinch a coin, "tuck your tail under," and brace your abs for an imaginary punch. Expect a mighty "Ouch!"

Having learned that extra tension adds power, now find a way of maximizing that tension. One technique is bracing, or tightening up your muscles before the load is placed upon them.

A good arm-wrestler loads all his muscles with high-strung tension before the ref yells "Go!" A great arm-wrestler will load even before gripping up with his or her opponent. And an amateur, who waits for the referee's command to pull before turning on his biceps, will get pinned without even knowing what hit him.

Conduct another experiment: Get down in a pushup position, elbows locked. Have a Comrade push down on your shoulders a few times. Note how heavy the pressure feels. Now brace yourself, flex your whole body, and have your buddy push again with the same amount of force. This time, you won't even notice the pressure!

The lesson to learn is to brace yourself while the bell is still in the air, not when it hits you. Houdini could take anyone's punch, if he was prepared for it. He died when he got struck without warning.

The body-hardening technique, or controlled striking of the target muscles, especially those of the core, will also come in handy.

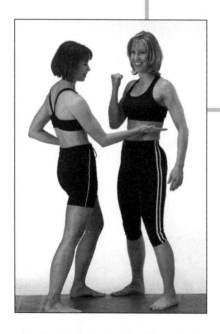
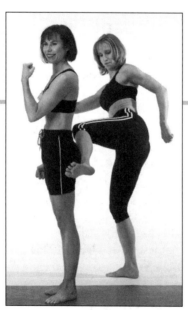
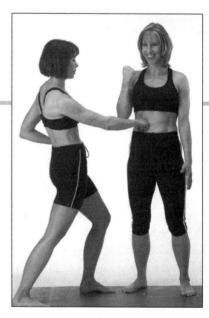

How can you get the most out of your press? While putting the least amount of distress on your shoulder, you must start the movement with your working shoulder maximally pressed down, away from your ears—the opposite of a shrug—and your elbow pushed down as low as it can go. At the same time, pull your elbow slightly in toward your belly button. This maneuver from the arsenal of Russian weightlifters—the so-called *obtyazhka*—prestretches the delts. As a result, you will be stronger. Starling's law states that a prestretched muscle has more "oomph."

First practice pressing your bell with another hand over the pressing hand. You'll notice that the press will have an interesting path that pulls in toward the center of your body. This will work your upper pecs in addition to your shoulders.

- **Maximally tighten your body on impact when you are cleaning the kettlebell.**

- **Start the press with your working shoulder maximally pressed down—the opposite of a shrug—and your elbow pushed down as low as it can go.**

- **At the same time, pull your elbow slightly in toward your belly button.**

- **First practice pressing your bell with another hand over the pressing hand.**

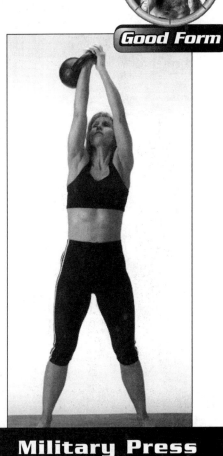

Good Form

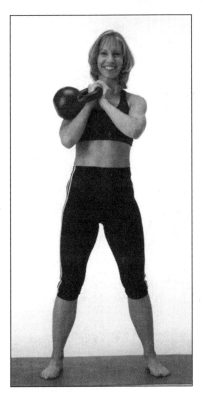
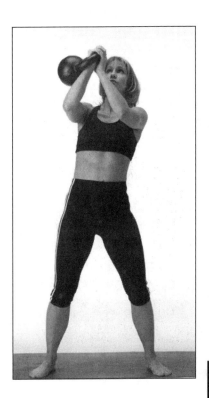

Military Press

What if I want to work my pecs more?

Optional Technique

Try this unique kettlebell floor press: Lie on your back, and carefully take a kettlebell in your left hand with the help of your right. Stick your slightly bent right arm under a couch, palm up, to anchor yourself. Both of your feet will be facing the couch, as if you are walking. Your feet should be spread as wide apart as your flexibility allows, the left leg atop the right one and closer to the couch.

Press your left shoulder into the floor. Now, thanks to the body roll away from the kettlebell, you can perform chest presses with a range of motion every bit as long as what you would get on a bench.

Inhale, tighten up, and push the KB up in a wide arc. If you let the kettlebell come to the centerline before you have reached the lockout, you will be working your triceps more than your chest.

Carefully lower the weight until your elbow rests on the floor. Take care not to slam your elbow into the floor; control the movement all the way down. To maximize pec recruitment, flare your elbow and let the bell fall out somewhat, as if you are about to do a fly.

You may perform the twisted floor press with your palm facing forward, as in the barbell bench press, or with your palm facing in.

Look at the photos and observe that the hip is slightly kicked over to the side to allow being positioned straight under the bell. It's time you understood that pressing a heavy weight overhead while standing totally upright is a fantasy. Even a so-called certified personal trainer cannot defy Newtonian physics. The downward pressure of the weight must be projected over your feet—at least if you don't feel like toppling over. Maybe you can keep your waist relaxed and upright and still make it—if you are pressing a Malibu Ken and Barbie pink dumbbell with your little finger sticking out. But when the iron adds up, the scenario changes.

• **Your hip might slightly kick over to the side to get positioned straight under the kettlebell.**

Military Press

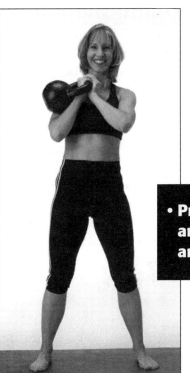

Realize that displacing your hips sideways doesn't give you an excuse to lean back. That would be plain bad news for your back. Note that although D.C.'s upper body tilts back slightly under a 36-pound kettlebell, an intense ab, glute, and thigh contraction keeps her back strong.

• Protect your back with an intense ab, glute, and thigh contraction.

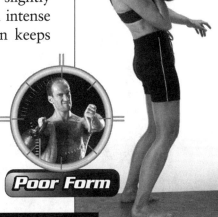

Poor Form

• You may not lean back.

A stable platform to push from

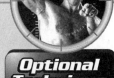

Optional Technique

A structure is only as strong as its foundation. That means wobbly legs are a recipe for disaster! So flex your quads and pull up your kneecaps when overhead pressing.

A one-legged kettlebell military press, practiced by Steve Maxwell, M.S., RKC, will help you learn this important skill. You will quickly learn that you won't success unless you pull up your groin muscles and flex your glute, like you did for the one-legged deadlift, and lock your knee and pull up your kneecap. Remember what this feels like for when you do standard presses on two feet.

Squeeze the kettlebell as you press it, and remember to keep your wrist tight. Make sure that the KB's handle rests on the meaty spot at the very base of your palm on the side of your little finger. When pressure stimulates the mechanoreceptors at that site, they send a command to the triceps to contract more intensely, a so-called *extensor reflex*.

Keep your shoulder pressed down as much as possible throughout the press. It may help to visualize that you're pushing yourself away from the weight, rather than pressing it up. Or concentrate on keeping your lat flexed. Flare it like a bodybuilder who's trying to impress you.

Military Press

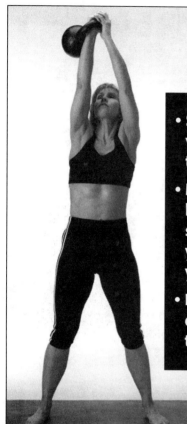

You should have taken a breath before you even cleaned the weight—75% of your lungs' vital capacity is optimal, according to Professor Arkady Vorobyev. Hold your breath and keep your abdomen pressurized until you fix the bell overhead. If you breathe with the kettlebell on your chest, you will lose tension.

- **Squeeze the kettlebell as you press it, and remember to keep your wrist tight.**

- **Make sure that the bell's handle rests on the meaty spot at the very base of your palm on the side of your little finger.**

- **Keep your shoulder pressed down as much as possible throughout the press.**

Obviously, if you have high blood pressure, a heart condition, or some other health concerns, this may not be an option. Ditto for full-body tension exercises, such as this one. Consult with your doctor on the breathing pattern most appropriate for you.

When you are exerting yourself, always contract your rectal sphincter, as if you are trying to stop yourself from going to the bathroom. (I explained the reasons behind this madness in *Power to the People!: Russian Strength Training Secrets for Every American.*)

Finish the lift slow and tight, and firmly lock out your elbow. Don't even bother to listen to the Nervous Nellies who tell you never to lock your joints! Leave them alone with their pencil-neck weights and hypochondria. Your joints need strengthening as much as your muscles, and locking out is the way to do it.

Let some air out, take some in, and head back to earth. If you are doing high-rep presses (which I don't recommend), you may exhale on the way down through pursed lips or a partially constricted throat.

- **Visualize that you are pushing yourself away from the weight rather than pressing it up.**

- **Keep your lat flexed, if you know how.**

- **You should have taken a breath before you even cleaned the weight.**

- **Hold your breath and keep your abdomen pressurized until you lock out the bell overhead. (If you have health concerns, follow your doctor's advice on breathing and tension.)**

Military Press

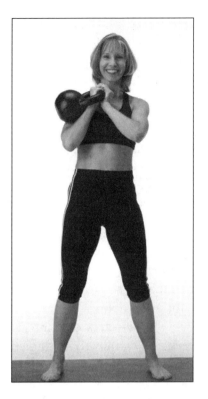

- **When you are exerting yourself, always pull up your pelvic floor.**

- **Finish the lift slow and tight, and firmly lock out your elbow.**

- **Let some air out, take some in, and head back to earth.**

- **If you are doing high-rep presses (which are not recommended), you may exhale on the way down through pursed lips or a partially constricted throat.**

Safer and more effective high rep presses

If you do more than a couple of military presses from your shoulders, your waist and the rest of your power base will lose its tightness. The results will be mediocre presses and back injuries. When you reclean the bell before each press, you are forced to brace your body to accept the shock. It's like loading a spring before the press. Make sure to press without any delay, or you will lose some tightness.

This business of "getting tight" is very important. An old-timer friend of mine, who started lifting at the Santa Monica Muscle Beach 50 years ago, tells of watching weightlifter David Ashman, famous in his day, as he practiced his jerks (quick lifts from the shoulders) with 500 pounds. Ashman couldn't clean that weight by himself. Instead of simply taking the barbell from the stands set up at his chest level, he had two guys, one on each end of the bar, help him clean the weight in a precisely synchronized and dangerous effort. Ashman understood that he could never get tight enough under a dead weight sitting in the rack. If he was willing to go to all the trouble with such huge poundage, believe that cleaning your kettlebell before pressing it is worth it. And if you choose to do more than 5 reps per set, it's almost a must. Besides, cleans-and-presses have great cardiovascular and fat-burning powers.

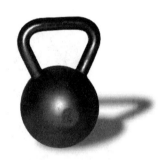

Optional Technique

Military Press

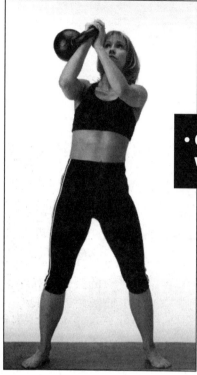

There is more to lowering a weight than meets the eye. In order to keep your shoulder in an antishrug, actively pull your elbow down—all the way to your navel. Quite literally, pull the bell down with your lat. Read all the instructions many times before tackling the weight; there are no minor points here.

• On the way down, actively pull your elbow down with your lat—all the way to your navel.

When you are ready to tackle the one-arm press, pay attention to the following very different groove. Start the press in an almost curl position. Don't press the bell straight up; your delts will have no leverage. Visualize pushing out with your elbow—sort of a lateral raise—while keeping your forearm vertical, rather than angled toward your head.

It's elementary mechanics, Watson. You will never press a heavy weight overhead unless you keep your forearm vertical. Consider almost overdoing it the other way: Push the weight away from your body almost to the point where it falls sideways. You will recruit more muscles in the effort, even your biceps.

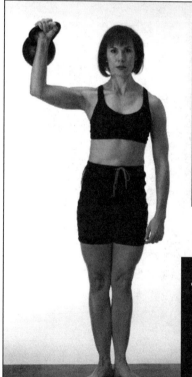

• The one-arm press has a different "groove."

• Start the press in an almost curl position.

As the bell is inching up, your hand will be gradually turning until it faces forward on the top. This is very similar to the Arnold Press, except that you will be locking your elbow on the top.

As the bell passes your head, lean forward against it and lock the weight out in the press behind your neck position. This will improve your shoulder flexibility and discourage you from leaning back. Keep pushing the bell even higher by making your arm long and rigid.

• Do not press the bell straight up; visualize pushing outward with your elbow—sort of a lateral raise—while keeping your forearm vertical.

Military Press

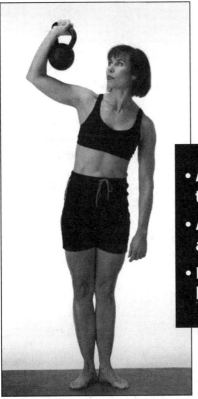

As the bell passes your head, lean forward against it and lock the weight out in the press behind your neck position. This will improve your shoulder flexibility and discourage you from leaning back. Keep pushing the bell even higher by making your arm long and rigid.

- **As the bell is inching up, your hand will be gradually turning until it faces forward on the top.**
- **As the bell passes your head, lean forward against it and lock the weight out in the press behind your neck.**
- **Keep pushing the bell even higher by making your arm long and rigid.**

As an option, you may keep your heels together, as shown. In fact, this "at attention" alignment is responsible for the name of the military press. Note that your body may have to tilt sideways to balance yourself under a heavier kettlebell. You will discover that squeezing your thighs together tight will increase your pressing power remarkably and stabilize your lower back.

- **Squeezing your thighs together tight will increase your pressing power remarkably and stabilize your lower back.**

Good Form

Military Press

Build muscle where it counts

The *From Russia with Tough Love* exercises will strengthen and firm your whole body without adding much muscle, and the muscle that you will gain will pleasantly flow with your curves. Expect a few pounds of dense, fat-burning meat on your upper and lower back. You will look great in a swimsuit and in a business suit.

Don't be surprised by this program's apparent lack of work for some muscles (such as the biceps). It's a fact that small muscles will take care of themselves once you take care of the big ones. Your biceps cannot help but get stronger and harder from all the swings and snatches you'll do. Ditto for the other small muscles. If you think your calves are lacking attention, consider skipping rope as a part of your *From Russia with Tough Love* routine—for instance, a kettlebell exercise, half a minute of rest, jump rope, half a minute of rest, and a kettlebell exercise.

Fill out in all the right places

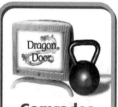

Comrades speak out on the dragon door.com forum

Re: Exrecondoc, Rob Lawrence, or Dano conflict? Between RKC & PTP
From: exrecondoc

As far as RKC' creating bulk, I will give you my personal experience. RKC' did cause me to loose bodyfat. You will not get chafing thighs from doing 50 snatches the way you will from doing 20-rep breathing squats. The only bulk I gained was in the upper back. You need never bulk up if you maintain dietary discipline. This is a great way to train. Don't fret about details; just enjoy it.

Re: Kettlebell testimonies
From: jdljon

In about 3 months, I have gained 10 pounds of solid muscle, especially upper-back and shoulders and lower-back muscles. I wasn't intentionally trying to gain, either. ... KB's work. They are a gift for life and vitality. Get 'em!!!

My results, up to this point
From: dogchild

I've lost size in my arms, but my arms are much harder. I think I had big, bloated bodybuilder-type muscle instead of hard, solid, functional muscle. Well, I've got it

now. I have "cuts" in my shoulders again for the first time in a long time. My traps are bigger. I seem to be compacting my physique, and I'm getting more muscular in a smaller package. Exactly what I wanted.

Re: Weight gain when KB-ing
From: blackrt

Although I have not gained but lost about 5 pounds on RKC', I have gained some mass, especially in my upper back and shoulders.

Re: Weight gain when KB-ing
From: drpower

I have had some weight loss, and my pants are looser around the waist now that the holidays are over. But I have gained mass between the shoulders and along the spine. I have worked this area with heavy rows and all sorts of stuff to no avail until now. I have also gained in the hamstring.

Re: Cardio suggestions
From: David C.

By the way, my wife likes the effect this workout has had on my physique, especially in the back and shoulders—something to think about.

Strengthen your legs and open your shoulders with the OVERHEAD SQUAT

Once your shoulder feels strong, flexible, and stable while doing the one-arm military presses, you should try the overhead squat. It's just like the front squat, except the kettlebell is held overhead in your straight arm. It's a good idea first to practice squatting to a box, as we did with other types of squats.

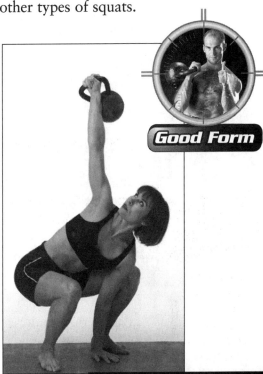

Good Form

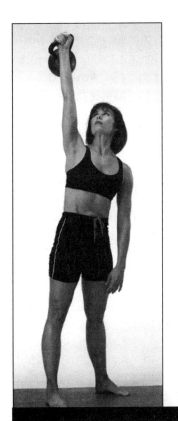

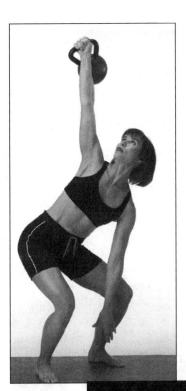

- **Keep your elbow completely locked and the whole length of your arm firm.**

- **Push up toward the ceiling with your straight arm; it will feel like you are elongating it.**

- **Keep your eyes on the kettlebell.**

- **Lean away from the kettlebell.**

- **Imagine "pulling your hips out of the sockets" as you are going down.**

- **Keep your reps very low—no more then 5, often less.**

- **Follow all of the other safe squat procedures discussed earlier.**

Overhead Squat

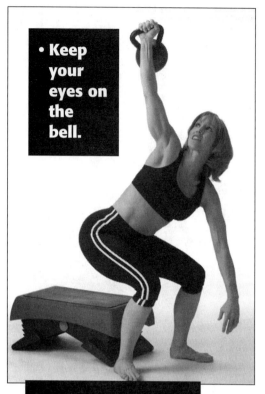

• Keep your eyes on the bell.

• It's a good idea first to practice squatting to a box.

The overhead squat imposes great demands on your shoulder flexibility and balance. Here are some tips to make your life easier: First, keep your elbow completely locked and the whole length of your arm firm. Push up toward the ceiling with your straight arm; it will feel like you are elongating it.

Second, keep your eyes on the bell.

Third, imagine "pulling your hips out of the sockets" as you are going down. To develop the proper feeling, lie on your back and raise your bent knees until they are perpendicular to the ground. Arch your lower back, push your chest out, and push your tailbone into the floor—just your tailbone, not your lumbar spine, as you would during crunches. There should be a gap in your lower back.

Spread your knees, inhale, and while arching your lower back as much as you can without discomfort, push your knees out, as if you're trying to push the walls apart. Don't just spread your knees; actively "pull your hips out of their sockets," so you feel like they have gotten longer. Do the same when you descend into a squat, and you'll be amazed at your squatting flexibility and control. Feel free to apply this technique to other kinds of squats.

Due to the rapidly building fatigue of the shoulder, you are advised to keep the reps very low in this drill—no more then 5, often less.

Look at the photos and note that Comrades Andrea and D. C. are leaning away from the kettlebell. Doing this will help you to stay in control. Eventually, once you are very flexible, you may try squatting with no sideways lean.

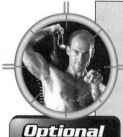

Optional Technique

An advanced challenge

You may practice this or any other KB drill that you have mastered with your eyes shut. Doing so will increase the difficulty of the exercise and improve your strength for obscure motor-learning reasons that I have explained in *Power to the People!: Russian Strength Training Secrets for Every American*. The standard protocol is to "go blind" every other set.

Overhead Squat

Mold a graceful and athletic body with the *TURKISH GETUP*

Few exercises will give you as much feeling of precise control as the Turkish getup. It feels like a yoga practice.

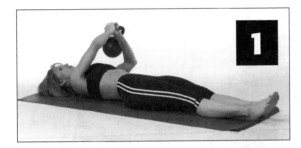

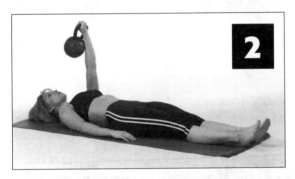

To begin, lie on your back. Carefully get your kettlebell up in your straight arm. Slowly and carefully (there is nothing ballistic about this drill!) roll away from the bell. Follow the rules of overhead squatting: eyes on the bell and so on. Stay tight, especially in your stomach, throughout the set. Taking shallow breaths will help you stay tight.

• **Follow the alignment rules of overhead squatting.**

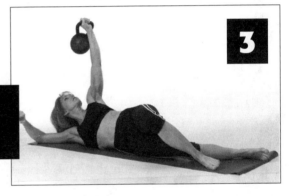

Think yourself strong

In a recent study (Ranganathan et al., 2001), the subjects increased their biceps strength by 13% in 12 weeks just by thinking about maximally flexing that popular muscle! Now it makes sense why you should treat your iron time as a practice rather than a workout. You can sum up effective strength training as *honing your skill in contracting your muscles harder.* Quoting Professor Thomas Fahey, "Skill is perhaps the most important element in strength." In Russian sports science, there is even a term—*skill strength*—and your date with iron is referred to as a lesson or a practice. So practice fresh and stop before your skill starts deteriorating.

Turkish Getup

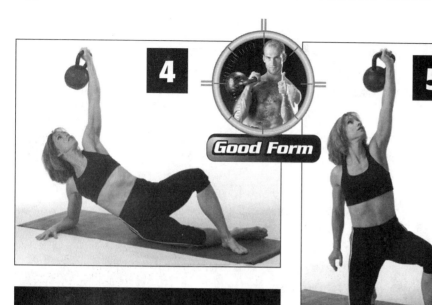

4   **Good Form**

5

6

- Stay tight, especially in your stomach, throughout the set.
- Take shallow breaths.
- Move smoothly.

Prop yourself up on your free elbow. Push yourself up and get on one knee. Carefully stand up.

Instead of kneeling, you may get up using the overhead squat shown below.

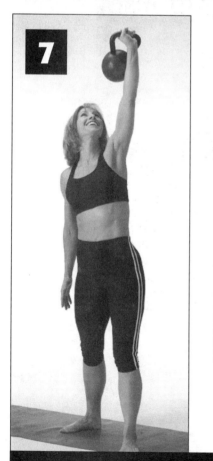

7

Turkish Getup

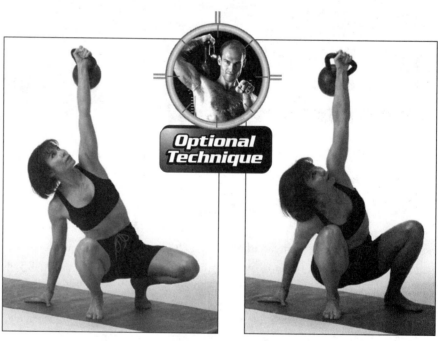

Optional Technique

Now go back down in reverse order. You may be surprised to find that going down us harder then standing up. As with the overhead squats, you are advised to keep your repetitions very low.

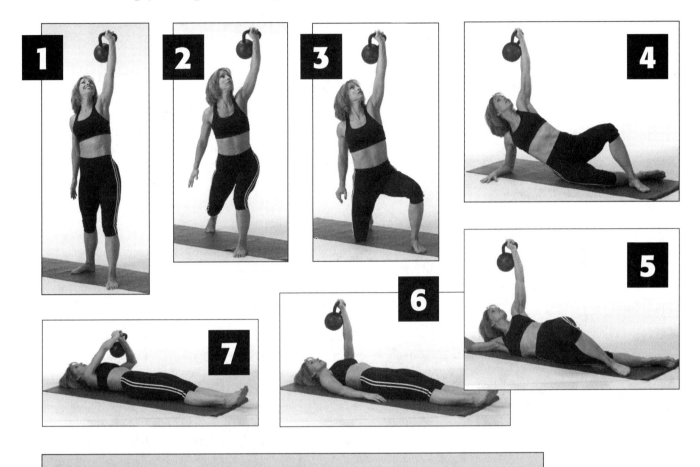

To work your abs more

Try this unique situp if your body is ready for it. Have your training partner hold your ankles in the starting position of the Turkish getup. Take a diaphragmatic breath, tuck in your tail by flexing your glutes, and press your lower back into the floor. Without help from your other arm, perform a controlled situp.

Literally push up with your straight arm (remember elongation?) to make the exercise safer and to better work your abs and other torso muscles, such as the serratus anterior.

Go up until you are sitting upright, the kettlebell overhead. Take another breath, and roll down on your hard, flexed glutes. Obviously, your stomach and back need to be in a decent shape before you try this overhead situp.

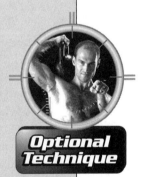

Optional Technique

Turkish Getup

Shed cellulite, get a hard butt, and enjoy the cardio workout of a lifetime with the SNATCH

Say no to fat and aerobics!

Through a mutual friend, WashingtonPost.com columnist Marty Gallagher, I had the pleasure of being introduced to Len Schwartz, M.D., the inventor of Heavyhands". He's a man who, at an age when most guys consider reaching for the remote to be heavy exertion, can knock off one-arm chins and other equally impressive feats. Len sports a GQ physique, to boot.

Dr. Schwartz conducted in-depth research at the Human Energy Laboratory, University of Pittsburgh, on the training effects of what he calls Panaerobic" exercise: where you combine hand weights with walking and various other forms of movement. He reported spectacular fat loss from this type of exercise and rightfully referred to his method as "the premier method for controlling body composition."

It makes sense that kettlebell lifting has the same effect. No guesses here: I have seen it time and time again in the Old Country, and it works just as well on this side of what used to be the Iron Curtain. Just see the testimonials in the sidebar.

The fat loss power of the kettlebell is explained by the extremely high metabolic cost of throwing a weight around combined with the fat-burning effect of the growth hormone that's stimulated by such exercise. Prominent strength and bodybuilding coach Charles Poliquin, explains it like this:

> Here's the idea: If you generate a lot of lactic acid during your weight-lifting sets, your body will then produce more growth hormone. Growth hormone helps your body release fatty acids from your fat cells, which you then use for energy. Result: You get muscle from lifting weights, and you lose fat. For most guys, the net result will be lost weight, without having to run a mile or take a single Spinning class. To make this work, though, you have to rethink the way you lift. . . . To generate enough lactic acid to promote fat loss, you have to extend your sets to about a minute, then rest for a minute, then move on to your next set. (Nobody said it was easier than aerobics.)

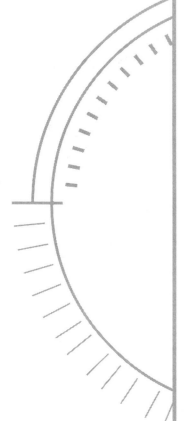

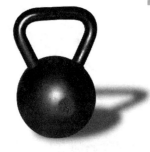

Burn fat without the dishonor of dieting and aerobics!

Steve
From: Mongo
I dumped the classic 1% bodyfat last week working with the KB.

Gosh darn it Andy68 (and Pavel)! You are right!
From: Margam
"Lose fat without the dishonor of dieting and aerobics." Because of elbow and knee tendonitis, I just did kettlebell swings everyday to give those joints a rest. So far it has worked great. Instead of taking a layoff from exercise altogether (which was what a lot of people were telling me to do) I made it a goal to do a 100 reps with my 1.5kg kettlebell. Not only is my tendonitis just about gone, but I have gotten leaner in the short time I have been doing this. For those of you looking to get leaner for the summer, give it a shot. Be careful with the volume at first. My lower back and hamstring muscles were very sore so I had to reduce the reps at first. I stuck with it and it is no longer an issue. Today I added chins, dips, and partial handstand pushups, and felt strong and pain free. Sometimes I think we make things too complicated. A simple exercise routine done consistently will work. Don't take my word for it. Just try swings, or cleans, or snatches everyday and see for yourself!

…Basically all I do is 1 or 2 arm swings till I get a 100 reps with as few breaks for rest as possible. It depends on how I feel that day on how many sets I can complete the 100 reps. Lately, for variety I have been doing cleans also. My best so far has been 2 sets -very tough for me! You can definitely trim some fat off. My diet has been very bad, but I can tighten up my belt 1 more notch! I am doing this every day, sometimes twice a day. I should warn you like Pavel warned me, be careful of too much volume at first. You can end up incredibly sore.

There's believing and then there's BELIEVING! Future kettlebellers please read.
From: Medic1
If anyone is still thinking about whether or not to take the plunge into kettlebelldom let me tell you a few things about my experiences with them. I have been working with k-bells for about 4 months now. For the first 3 months or so I was just tossing them around here and there getting used to them. I must admit the most appealing thing about them is that they are fun to work with, many will tell you that. Over time I became familiar with the lifts and swings…

Over the last month or so I began training with them in earnest. Mostly I was doing ballistics since I was trying to drop some body weight and working anywhere from 3-4 times a week for about 30 minutes. Then one day it happened. I was going out with my wife one day when she said, "Hey, you haven't worn those jeans for a while." I looked down and realized my mistake. I had a pair of jeans that used to fit really tight (Levi's 505's) laying in the drawer next to my regular jeans that fit comfortably (Levi's 560's). I had grabbed the tight jeans without realizing it and then couldn't tell the difference!

I was overjoyed! I was losing weight! So the next day at work I stepped onto the scales to see how many pounds I had lost. When I first got the k-bells I weighed 220 lbs. After "playing around" with them for 3 months I had gone up to 225 lbs. That day at work I weighted 227 lbs.

(Continued,)

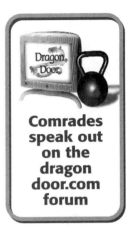

Comrades speak out on the dragon door.com forum

Re: Comrades, please tell your KB fat-loss stories
From: sebarnes
Been following Pavel's recommendations with a DB for 4 weeks. I've lost an average of 1% bodyfat per week, from about 20 to about 16. Love handles gone!

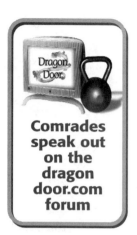

Comrades speak out on the dragon door.com forum

Re: Kettlebell testimonies
From: MoWeardslee

Oh, yeah . . . I also dropped about 20 pounds.

M/22/Printer repair guy/Lost about 75lbs o' flab KBing/NewHampshire. n/m
From: ComradeYojimbo

At home my wife pointed out that obviously my bodyfat percentage had gone down since my waist got smaller but my weight went up. Also she pointed out that my back was looking much more "V" shaped and muscular. Figures I would not see that since my back is behind me, but she noticed. And if she's happy I'm happy. Actually, she has also asked me to order her a kettlebell of her own so we can workout together.

Bottom line: These things work, people, no two ways about it… I have seen it for myself and I know this stuff works. And without intricate dieting or fancy supplements, although I'm sure that would enhance (speed up) the effect even more. Thanks Pavel, for a GREAT product!

One more story
From: JCannon

For almost 3 years, I have done personal training with a woman who has achieved average results. Then, 2 months ago, I started her on Power to the People! and worked in cycles of RKC' last month. She was literally firming up and slimming down before my eyes. She called the other day, bubbling and gushing over the phone that she was at a weight she hadn't been at for 15 years and wearing clothes she could only fit into before she had her teenage daughter! Me thinks the Party is a good place to be.

My results, up to this point
From: dogchild

I've been doing ballistic KBs—let me check my workout journal—I've been doing them since March 11. So, about 6 weeks. I immediately put on 3 pounds the first 2 weeks, as my body adapted to the swings. Soon, though, the weight started coming off. I'm 5 pounds down from where I started (8, if you count the muscle mass increase I got the first 2 weeks). My waist size is down an inch and a half.

This isn't with constant ballistic training, though. I took 10 days off for spring break and 4 days off because I was overtraining. So, I'd say these are results that you could get in about a month, month and a half of training. Also, watch your diet.

These explosive KB drills are making me svelte
From: Master Rinpoche

Last night, I didn't get home till late, and I had no groceries, and it was snowing. (Sounds like the beginning of one of my grandfather's stories). The only thing open close by was McDonald's, and my wife was yelling that she was hungry and wanted something quick.

I was starving and ate a Big Mac, super-size fries, a Coke, an apple pie, and a hot fudge sundae.

Weighed in this morning—expecting to have bloated out from the salt/fat/carbs nightmare I just ingested —and I had lost a couple pounds.

Now, I wouldn't keep eating like this every day, but it's nice to see I can abuse myself once in a while, as long as I exercise right. I like the tight, wiry strength I'm getting, too —even if my jujutsu mates don't.

KB burns lots of carbs
From: Mongo

Lessons Learned:

1. KB burns a deceivingly large amount of calories.

2. You should not restrict your intake as much as you might for some other fitness programs.

3. Things are not always what they seem.

4. KB is better for calorie burning than running.

5. PAVEL WAS RIGHT!!!!!

Kettlebells are . . .
From: primer

The way to go! The RKC' high-rep snatch workout is incredible. I got my pulse up to around 180 for about 20 minutes. I only started my RKC' cycle last week and was aching for 2 days afterward, but I did another one 2 days ago and I'm not as sore this time. I only worked out 2 days last week (because I was sore after the first workout), but I still lost a respectable amount of bodyfat.

Fat-loss report: Thanks Pavel and Party
From: Barry1001

After 5 months as a Party Member, I've lost 7 pounds of fat and gained 11 pounds of lean mass, and I can definitely feel and see it. I'm doing PTP [Power to the People] and RKC', plus running once or twice weekly. Diet is nothing special; try not to stuff myself with high fat; get enough protein and fruits and veggies. My thanks to Pavel and the Party.

Re: Good KB workout for fat loss
From: Master Rinpoche

I gotta say that the explosive drills in RKC' are the best thing I have ever done for fat loss. I'm building dense strong muscle and shedding fat like nobody's business.

Re: KB and appetite
From: Braveheart

I have noticed the same thing. Daily workouts of 10–15 minutes make me so hungry, but I am leaner and feel great. I was not heavy to start with, but people have remarked that I look thinner. Your body runs like 4 cylinders when you use KBs.

. . . Then did RKC
From: phv

After about 3 weeks of RKC' (mostly swings and under-leg pass, some push presses, jerks, and two-hand bottoms-up military presses), I tore up my pants doing push presses. (It was Halloween—didn't want to scare the trick-or-treating kids in my nasty workout clothes.) I had to go buy a replacement pair and was shocked to find 36" waist pants being too large —I had to get a 34" waist pair. All with no diet changes.

Fat loss redux—most mileage from a 1-pood KB?
From: Brian G

Six weeks of mostly KB workouts have dropped an inch off my waist and burned off a lot of fat.

Hacking fat off meat
From: craigN

In the last few months, I've hacked off about 25 pounds of lard without even cutting out the goodies or doing any special eating plan, simply by doing three RKC' workouts per week, each of which averages the equivalent of around 120 reps of 2-pood ballistics, floor to full overhead. I usually keep wheezing the whole workout (i.e., I keep the rest breaks relatively short).

Weird side-effect of RKC
From: rmonti01

Ever since starting the RKC' at Maxercise, I have been very pleased with the results, but they came with an interesting side-effect. I have a killer craving for steak whenever I am hungry. It's the only food that will satiate my appetite.

PROGRESS!!!
From: Fish

Comrades, it seems just like it almost happened overnight. It's insane! The K-bells are just melting my fat away, and I'm loving every minute of it. Look out single-digit bodyfat and visible abs! Here I come!!!

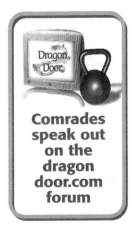

Comrades speak out on the dragon door.com forum

Re: Kettlebells
From: drc__

Let me warn potential K-bell buyers of a possible hidden expense. Yesterday, I blew some bucks buying new pants and belts; I had to drop the waistline a couple of inches.

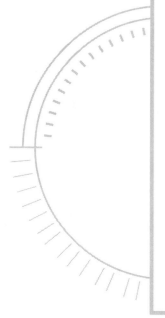

Why doesn't *From Russia with Tough Love* offer diet advice?

Two reasons. First, yours truly does not have the knowledge to write on the subject.

Second, as long as you follow a reasonable diet, you will lose plenty of fat—fast! —with kettlebells alone.

Let me add this caveat, however: Kettlebell training boosts your metabolism into overdrive, which means you will get very hungry. Don't give in to your mega-appetite; stick to your normal caloric consumption. Consider increasing the percentage of protein in your diet while keeping your calories static.

It's clear that Comrades D. C. Maxwell and Andrea Du Cane have developed a winning formula for themselves, with both their exercise and eating habits. I asked them to share their personal regimens with you:

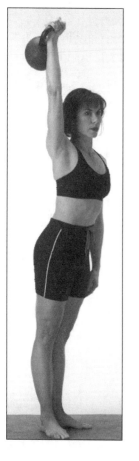

Comrade Andrea's Tough Love Diet Plan

Attaining and maintaining a healthy and fit body is the goal of many people. The way to achieve this goal is through a combination of exercise and diet. This book, *From Russia With Tough Love*, addresses the first part of the equation. I would like to take a moment and talk about the second part, diet and nutrition.

When I talk about diet, I am not referring to just restricting what one eats. This is a common mistake that many people make. The key is to eat the right kinds of foods for your particular body, metabolism and lifestyle. It also includes adding the right kind of supplements to help make up for what the food lacks in nutrients as well as assisting the body to help you achieve your fitness goals.

I believe in balance. A healthy balance of the right amount and kind of exercise and a balance in what one eats. I don't believe in "fad" diets or completely eliminating a food group. Unless one has an actual food allergy or it goes against your ethical belief system, there is no good reason from a health perspective to eliminate a particular food group.

As I said before, diet and nutrition is a very personal thing. What works for me may not work for you.

First of all, I try to exercise 3–6 times a week. It varies depending on my work schedule, personal life and energy level. I vary my workouts as much as possible. I may do an advanced step-aerobics class 3 times a week and 3–4 kettlebell workouts of various lengths and intensities. Some weeks I hardly workout at all, some weeks I workout nearly everyday. This works for me because I am constantly changing what and when I put my body through a workout. My eating and diet vary almost as much.

One of the most important things I do that enables me to keep a lean body even during the weeks when I don't workout much, is eating enough protein. I ALWAYS have some form of whey protein within an hour of exercising. Instead of a protein drink, I add whey protein to goat's yogurt then add a high-fiber, unsweetened cereal. I might add some nuts and raisins as well. I find this fills me up and sustains me through till dinner. I should mention that most of my workouts are in the morning or around noon.

I start my day with a glass of orange juice, to which I add L-Glutamine powder and a packet of Emergen-C. This is when I take my amino acids, vitamins etc. Then during the morning, if I feel hungry I'll have some fresh whole fruit, a green-juice drink or some nuts and seeds.

After my workout, I'll have my "protein/cereal". During the afternoon, if I get hungry I'll have some more fruit and nuts or a protein bar. Sometimes I might mix some protein powder into water or milk for a little more protein. For dinner I eat anything I feel like. I always try to have a balance of vegetables and protein.

This is not to say I'll not have some Black Bean Chili Chips, or a desert.

I treat myself when and if I want to. Thanks to increasing my protein and thanks to some of my supplements, I don't have the cravings I used too. I don't beat myself up if I have an ice cream cone, or feel like I'm constantly denying myself things I want.

I am going to list some of the supplements that I use regularly and that I think are very beneficial:

Whey Protein Powder: Helps to rebuild muscle after workouts, maintains lean body mass, boosts the immune system and protects against cancer and free radicals.

L- Glutamine (peptide is best): Reduces fatigue, improves exercise endurance, boosts growth hormone secretion, reduces lactic acid buildup, has an anti-catabolic effect, maintains healthy gastrointestinal tract, combats hypoglycemia, reduces sugar cravings. 2 –10 grams before exercise or bed. Best taken on empty stomach.

Acetyl-L-Carnitine or L-Carnitine: Acetyl-Carnitine is more easily absorbed in the blood. Increases cellular energy. Assists the transport of fat into the mitochondria to produce the cellular energy ATP. Increases metabolism resulting in fat-burning. 2- 4 capsules daily 500mg each. Best taken on empty stomach with juice or water.

L-Tyrosine: Increases mental energy and elevates the mood. It is a precursor of the neurotransmitters dopamine, norepinephrine, epinephrine and the thyroid hormones. 500-1000mg in the morning or afternoon.

Taurine: Boosts cardiac output and metabolic processes, is involved with glucose uptake. 1-4 gms daily.

CLA: Reduces body fat while maintaining lean muscle mass. Increases basal metabolic rates. Decreases fat storage. 3-5 capsules daily.

Co Q-10: Is a dynamic antioxidant, which protects both the mitochondria and the cell membrane against oxidative damage. It is essential for the respiratory cycle of the cell and generates ATP, the cell's energy. 30mg-100mg best taken with some fat.

Alpha Lipoic Acid: Is a potent antioxidant, boosts glutathione levels and is involved in generating energy from food and oxygen in the mitochondria. 250mg am and pm.

EFAs (blend of omega 3's, 6's & 9's) or Flax seed oil: Building blocks of nerve cells and cell membranes. Reduces risk of cardiovascular disease, lowers bad cholesterol and elevates HDL levels, reduces arthritic inflammation and pain, good for common skin disorders such as eczema. Can be taken either as an oil (1-2 Tbls. once or twice a day), or capsules, 2 capsules 2-3 times daily.

Green tea (either as a tea or extract), Neutralizes cancer-causing agents, protects cells against mutation, protects against free-radical damage, reduces blood glucose, gentle stimulant.

Vitamin complex (may want extra B vitamin & at least 400mg of E)

Vitamin B's (75-100mg)

Vitamin C: (1000mg) (Emergen-C effervescent packets mixed in O.J.)

MSM: Good for all connective tissue, joints, skin.

Glucosamine/chondroitin: Healthy joints.

Coral Calcium/magnesium: Relaxes muscles, builds bones, balances blood pH.

Enzymes: Essential for good food digestion and absorption, can also be used between meals to help reduces muscle soreness.

I also use a number of herbs that are good for a variety of things. Ginseng, ginkgo, ephedra (not for long term use or for some people).

Listen to your body. Don't rely on scales, look in a mirror and see how your cloths fit. Pay attention to how eating certain foods make you feel. There is wisdom in the old Chinese proverb "Eat when you're hungry and sleep when you're tired". Sometimes the simplest things are the most effective. Remember it's not just about fitness it's about health. Finding what's right for you, is the key to a healthy and fit body!

As for her eating habits, D. C. Maxwell swears by Ori Hofmekler's *Warrior Diet* program. Like Andrea, D.C.'s training regimen has evolved from a wide range of experimentation, experience and styles of exercise:

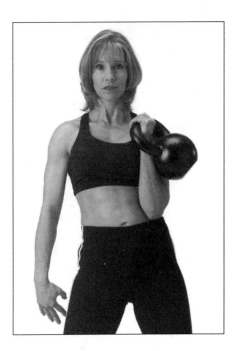

When Pavel requested that I write a few words about training, specifically women's training, I drew a blank. What did he want? What could I possibly have to say that hasn't been said before and besides, I'm really busy. And so the weeks rolled by with me being busy and Pavel being very patient. But this week I am a guest in someone else's house, in Rio de Janeiro, so far away from home, I'm in another hemisphere. I wake up and there is nothing I really have to do. Forget not having to go to work, it's even better than that. No children to direct, no clothes to wash, no house to clean no car to gas up, no pets to feed .....I wonder if I'm going to get to train today? Wait a minute. Maybe I do have something to say about training for women. After all, I do happen to be one. One who had trained for decades, through many phases, single, married, pregnant, not working at all, working too hard, training for competition, not training for anything in particular. Now that I think of it, I'm a freaking authority. I must be one of the world's foremost experts on the subject. But before my head swells too large, I must remind myself. Me and about a gazillion other women who work, have children and otherwise fit 10 lbs of stuff into a 5 lb bag every single day as a matter of course.

Like most women over the age of 30, I have seen it all and done most of it. I have seen fitness trends come and go and come again. I have seen the same concepts, from the right on to the way off, recycled, repackaged, and resold to a naive and often lazy public who wants to trust and believe, by an industry that is willing to lie. I have seen the pendulum swing back and forth enough times that sometimes I don't even point it out when it happens. But before I sound jaded, let me amend my original statement to say, I have seen it all and done most of it but still I get jazzed when someone shows me the same good idea in a different way. Because it's hard to come up with good ways, therefore, an incredible temptation to appeal to what people want to hear.

I have been active in sports for most of my life. I started competing in the 8 & under division of the neighborhood swim team and through my school years competed in gymnastics, field hockey and lacrosse. I have competed in a multitude of sports on every level from local to international.

Working out remained simple for me as long as I was single and young, even when I got married, it was simple. Youth was my trainer and youth forgives a multitude of sins. Because I had fairly good genetics, as long as I was very active, and watched my diet, things were fine. And it was easy to stay active because I had the time. Then I had my first child. My body changed. Then my husband and I started our own business. I had a second child. We added a business. I realized that my business education was incomplete so I went back to school part time. I fell in love with the sport of Brazilian Jiu-Jitsu and began serious training for competition.

My workouts evolved along the same lines as my life. I had enjoyed group exercise like step aerobics, but now I really didn't have the time. But I had to figure something out because my body wouldn't lie. It was just as obvious when I didn't work out as when I did. Did I mention that the business my husband and I started was a personal training facility? But I was working, not working out. We specialized in the 30 minute circuit style strength training session. The women flocked to us, mostly married working women who needed to fit some kind of training into the course of their workday because as soon as they went home they began the second shift of cooking, homework, preparing themselves and their children for the next day. Most of them, during the pre-training consultation never mentioned fun as a criterion of their workout. To a woman, they wanted to look and feel better, and they wanted to cut to the chase. Even if they had unrealistic expectations and crazy ideas about diet, by the end of 30 minutes every one of them was very clear about the relationship between strength training and real results that enhance every aspect of their lives, now and in the future. Train to live, don't live to train. I was selling fitness to myself in hundreds of incarnations. And the more we honed the workouts, the more efficient we made them, the more successful our facility, Maxercise became.

As for me, I have become the sultan of speed. I developed the Fitness Logic™ training system, which embraces many different protocols, but stays true to a brief, safe and productive format. And I still get jazzed by the new ideas and the new twists on old favorites, even ones that are from a different time and place, like Pavel's kettlebells. I depend on my husband, Stephen, to cast his net over the world of training, sift the information through his 25 years of knowledge and experience, discard what is dangerous or inefficient and fit the golden nugget of what's left into some coherent order and structure. Fast. The first time I looked at a kettlebell I wanted no part of that cannonball with a suitcase handle. I had no idea what was to come of this association. Before I knew it, my workouts consisted solely of kettlebell exercises with a few bodyweight movements thrown in.

The last workout request I made before I departed on this trip was worded like this, "I've got 15 minutes. Kick my butt." In retrospect, I see that I gave myself more time than was necessary. In just 12 minutes, Stephen put me through a kettlebell workout that kicked my butt, cleaned my clock and otherwise accomplished the mission. After decades of work on machines, I am awestruck by how a simple cannonball with a suitcase handle can produce the results that I have experienced. When people I haven't seen for a year comment, " I've never seen your arms looking so good" I know for sure that I'm on to something. When people I don't know suggest that I spend 2 hours a day working out, I smile. Fifteen minutes, 2 or 3 times a week is all I can steal, but it's enough because of the incredible efficacy of a kettlebell workout.

But for this week, I am living in my friend's world. Two days ago I accompanied him to his gym. This gym is famous in Rio as a serious gym for fighters only, and he is one of them. Everyone's face I already knew from magazines. Every one of them performed their version of a hard core strength and conditioning workout and every workout seemed to take about 2 hours. This works for them because their lives between fights consist mostly of training and recovering. Being the only woman in the place, and a foreign one at that, I tried not to call attention to myself. I quietly went to an unpopulated corner and performed my own workout, an ascending chin and push-up ladder, followed by a descending dumbbell swing ladder (they had no kettlebells), and then partner ab work with the help of my friend. I noticed the faces of some of the fighters who were all pretending not to be looking, but there were a couple of open jaws. How could I be finished already? How could a woman work out that intensely and finish that fast? I smiled to myself. Guys, if you haven't noticed, I'm a woman. What that means is that I regularly fit 10 lbs of stuff into a 5 lb bag. And I'm a freaking authority on women's fitness training.

Make your fat go into a nuclear meltdown!

If your fat loss has flatlined, try this evil routine developed by RKC-certified instructor and Green Beret veteran Bill Cullen.

The program that Comrade Bill has implemented at the academy of one of the federal agencies where he is an instructor is deceptively simple: Do 50 kettlebell snatches or swings, 25 with one arm and then 25 with the other. Then immediately jog one-quarter of a mile or around a stadium.

Do not run—jog! The idea is to let your heart rate come back halfway to normal before doing the next set of snatches. Think of your jog as an active rest, not a race.

Next, do 40! Jog. 30! Jog. 20! Jog. 10! Jog. Walk.

By now, you will be dead meat—but much leaner dead meat!

Of course, you may tweak the sets, reps, and distances to suit your needs and level of conditioning. Just keep in mind the proven formula in all this: supersetting sets of 10 snatches with 1 minute of jogging.

Be warned: This program is extremely demanding, and you must be in top health and shape to take it on! Even so, you'll still likely cough up a hairball on this nuclear fat burner!

Optional Technique

Try this fat burner if you dare!

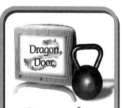

Comrades speak out on the dragon door.com forum

Marathon kettlebell training
From: Legbelu1

I don't know if anyone has ever tried this, but I just wanted to share something that I do with the KBs that's rather torturous but great for cardiovascular and muscle endurance (as if anything you do with KBs doesn't help that). I alternate workouts so that every other workout, I set it up this way: I take the Kettlebell and start doing whatever exercise that floats my boat for a minute, and then I switch to another exercise without putting the KB down. I continue doing a different exercise per minute without putting the KB down for 10 minutes; sometimes I boost it up and do up to 16 minutes—that's the most I've ever done like this. I tell you, ever since I've started working the kettlebells like this, my cardio is unbelievable and my overall endurance has skyrocketed.

Technically, a snatch is an uninterrupted smooth lift from the ground (we allow a swing back though) to the lockout overhead. You can think of the snatch as a clean to the point above your head. Don't even think about taking on the snatch until you have mastered one-arm swings, cleans, and military presses!

Start as if you are doing a swing or a clean. Keep pulling with your hips, and keep the bell fairly close to your body. Finally, let the bell flip over safely (remember the clean lessons) while taking a knee dip to help to dissipate the shock. It's generally not a good idea to swing the kettlebell in a wide arc around your hand because you will have to dip more to absorb the shock.

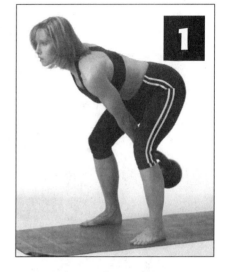

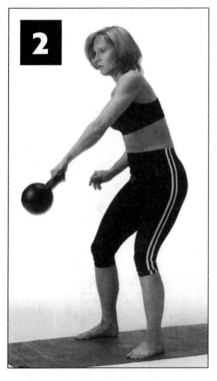

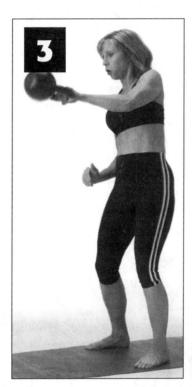

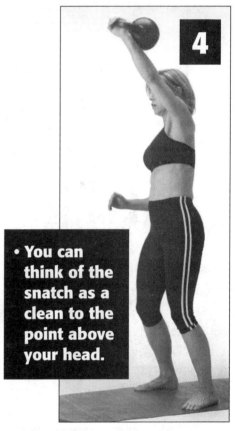

• You can think of the snatch as a clean to the point above your head.

• **Don't even think about snatching until you have mastered one-arm swings, cleans, and military presses.**

• **Start as if you are doing a swing or a clean.**

• **Keep pulling with your hips, and keep the bell fairly close to your body.**

• **Let the bell flip over safely overhead (remember the clean safety lessons) while taking a knee dip to help to dissipate the shock.**

Snatch

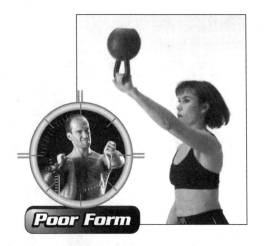

Poor Form

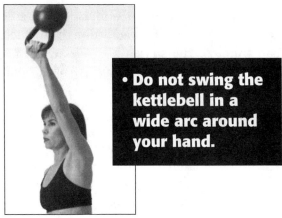

• Do not swing the kettlebell in a wide arc around your hand.

Finish in a strong stance with the bell locked overhead.

Now, you have two choices. One is to let the kettlebell freefall to the starting point behind your legs in a nearly straight arm, the swing style. The other is to softly, with a knee dip, lower the bell to your shoulder and drop it from there.

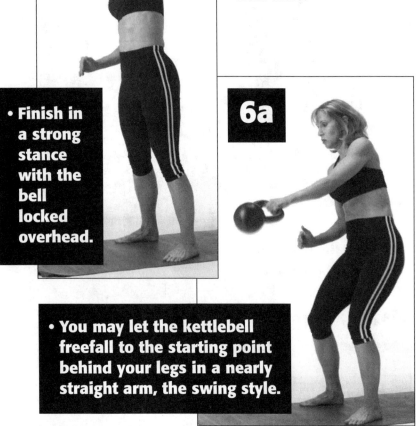

5

• Finish in a strong stance with the bell locked overhead.

• You may let the kettlebell freefall to the starting point behind your legs in a nearly straight arm, the swing style.

6a

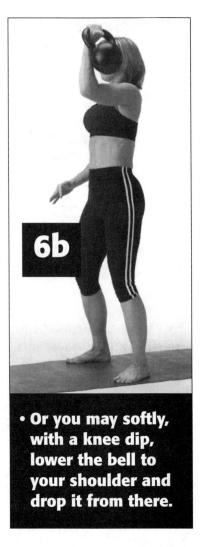

6b

• Or you may softly, with a knee dip, lower the bell to your shoulder and drop it from there.

Snatch

Follow the safety rules you learned with swings and cleans. When you drop the KB, don't let it pull you forward; stay back on your heels to decelerate the falling weight with your hamstrings.

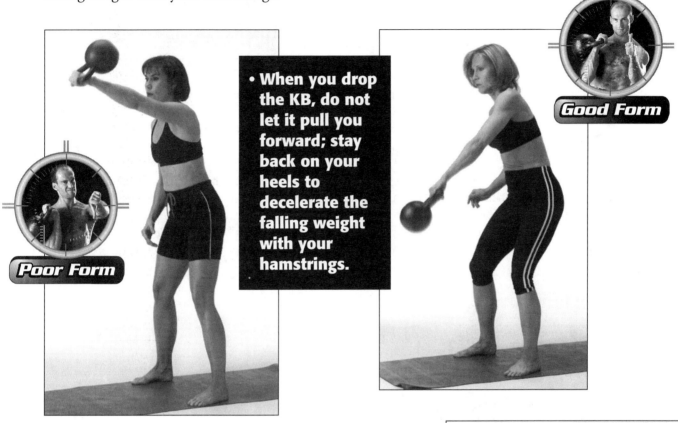

- When you drop the KB, do not let it pull you forward; stay back on your heels to decelerate the falling weight with your hamstrings.

Poor Form

Good Form

Enjoy!

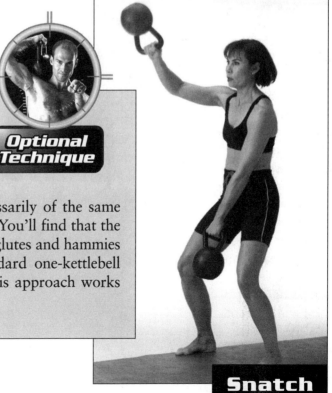

Optional Technique

If you insist on pulling with your shoulder instead of your hips . . .

Try this: Hold another kettlebell, not necessarily of the same weight, between your legs as a dead weight. You'll find that the added weight quickly forces you to put your glutes and hammies to work. Now, when you go back to standard one-kettlebell snatches, you'll clearly see the difference. This approach works for fixing your cleans, too.

Snatch

The kettlebell snatch—safer and more foolproof than most

Unlike the squat and many other exercises, the kettlebell snatch does not impose prohibitively strict requirements on spinal alignment and hamstring flexibility. If you are squatting with a humped-over back, you are asking for trouble. KB snatches let you get away with having a slightly flexed spine, probably because your connective tissues absorb shock more effectively when loaded rapidly. Your ligaments have wavy structures. A ballistic shock—as long as it is of a reasonable magnitude—is absorbed by these "waves," which straighten out like springs.

But if you keep the load on the ligament for more than a fraction of a second, the slack gets pulled out of the ligaments and predisposes them to tearing. That's why you have no business jerking your weights when performing grinding-type drills like deadlifts. Your ligaments may absorb the initial impulsive loading by losing their "waves," but by the time you get the bar to your knees, you will be ready for the emergency room.

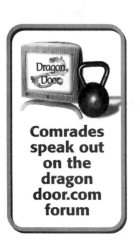

Comrades speak out on the dragon door.com forum

Snatch and nothing but the snatch

One-arm snatch only?

From: eklam

I love doing one-arm snatches. They are the only exercise I have done for about 3 weeks now, and the muscular and cardio benefits are amazing. I am currently doing 100 reps with each arm 4 times a week, alternating between the 1 and 1.5 pood on different days.

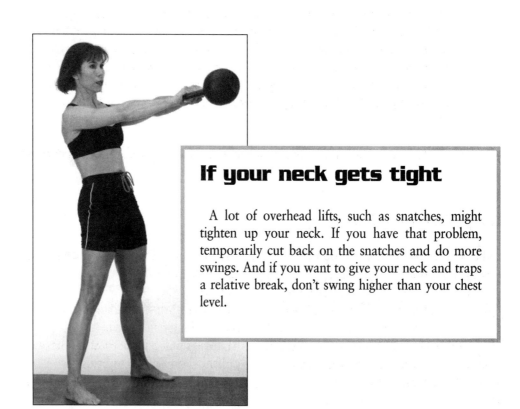

If your neck gets tight

A lot of overhead lifts, such as snatches, might tighten up your neck. If you have that problem, temporarily cut back on the snatches and do more swings. And if you want to give your neck and traps a relative break, don't swing higher than your chest level.

Snatch

Supercharge your heart and lungs without aerobics

One of the effects of Dr. Schwartz's *combined* exercise was a remarkable decrease in the trainees' heart rates—even the experienced runners whose RPMs had stabilized decades ago. As for the untrained people, their resting heart rates plummeted by 25 beats per minute after only 5 weeks of training! Dr. Schwartz's own motor beats a bare 35 beats per minute. Performing high-rep kettlebell drills have the same effect.

I recall a trip when my wife, Julie, and I drove from across the fruited plain to California. When we were in the mountains and the deserts, we saw dozens of minivans with lousy 4-cylinder engines stalled on the side of the road, waiting to get towed. Meanwhile, the V-8s cruised by without overheating. By the same token, someone with a high heart rate is at risk of "overheating," while both research and common sense suggest that a slower heart rate is a healthier heart rate.

Dr. Schwartz explains it like this:

A slow heart rate is a more effective heart-muscle supplier and safer than a fast heart. Why? Because the heart muscle fibers receive their oxygen-rich blood *between beats*; essentially, a slower hear rate means more opportunity for the heart itself to receive life-giving oxygen. If you choose a fast, sedentary heart rate over a slower trained one, you're also opting for a dangerously fast heart if you should forget yourself long enough to chase a bus!

So consider yourself warned by the author of *The Heavyhands Walking Book!*

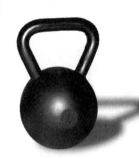

Beyond aerobics

KBs deliver fat loss, cardio gains
From: S Justus

In 6 weeks of training with KBs as my primary exercise, I lost 1.5 inches off my waist and stayed the same weight, so I lost fat and replaced it with muscle. My resting heart rate went from 60 to 52. It had been stuck at 60 for years, regardless of whatever sort of cardio training I did.

My protocol was pretty simple: one day emphasizing snatches and/or clean-and-jerks, followed by a day emphasizing presses, 5–6 days a week.

Is this the "What the hell effect" COM. Rob mentioned?
From: Pietro

Cuz that's what I said this morning while doing an intense 20-minute RKC.

I always pull on my HRM for these short pukers, even though my muscles were giving out and I was getting dizzy. I just couldn't get my heart rate above 180 for the life of me! When I first started RKC', I swear my heart rate hit 180 just picking up the weight.

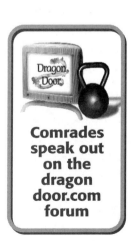

Comrades speak out on the dragon door.com forum

Snatch

Beyond aerobics (continued)

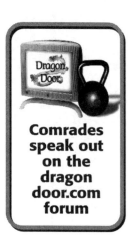

Comrades speak out on the dragon door.com forum

An interesting encounter with the treadmill...
From: dogchild

I had an interesting encounter with the treadmill today and I ran my first 6.5 minute mile... Why? I think the high volume of swings & snatches that I've been doing probably has something to do with it... I love my little ball of iron. Showed it to some more of my friends, and now they think I'm crazier than ever.

Re: Be totally honest with me—KBs or DBs?
From: craigN

I am not a runner, but the snatches and swings have put a real zip in my end of martial arts workout hill sprints and made my short-term wind like it was 30 years ago.

Re: K-bell result?
From: Mike Rinaldi

Thanks, Pavel!!! Also, all those reps helped normalize what was becoming a dangerously high blood pressure.

One month of KB's and heart BPMs
From: X-celsior

I've been doing KB's for about 1 and a half months now. Only about 3 weeks of serious practice. My back is finally pain free after about a year of on-and-off pain. My bench, deadlift, squat, etc. have all improved to some degree from nothing but KB's. My heart rate was already low from a lot of cycling, around 50 beats per minute. After these last 3 weeks of 6-day/week KB's, my heart rate is down to a low of 45. That's surely going to help when cycling season rolls back around next year.

I'm concentrating mostly on high-rep swings. To me, when done fast, they are harder than snatches. They're also a lot easier on my hands. My long days are

Mon, Wed, Fri, Sat. I usually total about 200+ reps/arm. I use mostly the 1-pood bell, but about one-fourth is with the 1.5-pood bell. I prefer to use the lighter bell for more volume.

My heavy/short days are Tues and Thurs. On these days, I use mainly the 1.5- and 2-pood bells.

I can't wait to see where my future training goes with the KB's.

Re: Series of questions for PAVEL and anyone else—KBs really that great???
From: Dano

Kettlebells aren't great—they are superb! You will be shocked and amazed, I guarantee. I think they improve your lung capacity more then running, plus you build crazy strength and agility at the same time, not to mention the endurance of a machine. I helps me chain sawing all day long.

KB vs. Tae Bo
From: sebarnes

Now, this is going to be embarrassing, but I have to admit that I enjoy doing Tae Bo tapes with my wife. The advanced ones, hitting a heavy bag, offer a decent sweat, and the time with the Better Half is great. But something interesting happened yesterday. It was the first time after several weeks of getting back to Tae Bo. My wife had been treadmilling faithfully, and we'd run on the track a bit, but I'd been KB'ing 5–6 days a week for the past 3 weeks and wondered how the Tae Bo would feel. Usually, we work hard enough (hitting a heavy bag for an hour is tough—even if only to an aerobics tape) for both of us to stop and gasp from time to time. Well, my wife was wiped out, and I was GRINNING through 90% of it. Only some of the small-muscle floor exercises taxed me at all! About all I can say is: Pavel, if you don't do a "KB Work-Along" tape for the general market, someone else is going to and will get rich doing it. Your methods are, quite simply, superb.

Re: Kettlebells cardio carryover?
From: matoyamazeki

Definitely, some major carryover. I used to run 3 miles a day in a morning and evening session of 1.5 miles each for about a year and a half. I usually only run about once or twice a week now and use KBs as my main cardio. I definitely felt a major increase in my wind. I can go out and crush 3–5 miles easily. Sometimes I run 2 miles and then come home and snatch a 45-lb dumbbell 50x. Can't wait till Xmas when my wife promised me a KB!

Re: Kettlebells cardio carryover?
From: Legbelu1

I can tell you that after a month of doing KB lifts, but done with a dumbbell, I was glad with the cardio carryover. I did them 2 to 3 times a week and saw increases in cardio performance after the first 3 workouts. I hit the bag and wrestle. I didn't hit the bag or wrestle for about 2 weeks but kept doing the KB stuff, and when I went back to it, I actually had more gas in the lungs, I didn't have to breathe as hard and wasn't as tired cardiowise, and I felt like I could keep my strength going for prolonged periods of time. KBs definitely had a carryover in my case.

Re: Kettlebells and running
From: little bear

I will just post my experience. Usually run 3x per week, 8-km route with 1,100-ft hill. (I live in the mountains.) Buddy who I run with and I are about the same speed. I stop running for 5 weeks and do nothing but kettlebells, 5x per week, with grinding one day, high-rep snatches 1-2-3-4-5-6-7-8-9-10-9-8-7-6-5-4-3-2-1 each arm, and clean-and-jerks, and under-the-leg pass the following day. My buddy keeps running for

those 5 weeks. We just went last week for a run, and I power past and sprint the last 200 vertical feet to the top of the hill. In other words, I kicked. I don't really understand why, but that is my experience. I believe that high-rep snatches and clean-and-jerks do build a lot of leg power as well as strengthen the tendons and ligaments from the ballistic forces. This must in turn give my stride that extra springy endurance that translates into faster running??

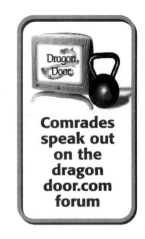

Comrades speak out on the dragon door.com forum

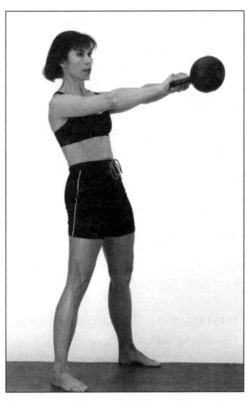

Pavel—KB routine
From: Gediminai

I love KB's! I have lost 16 pounds in the last four weeks since I started the KB lifts. Also, I haven't jogged in 2 weeks, and last night I went jogging after my KB workout. At the end of the course that I run, there is a big hill. Before KB's, I was dying at the beginning of the hill and a complete goner at the top. Last night, I threw the hill aside like a little pink plastic dumbbell!!!

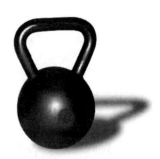

Combination exercises

Optional Technique

Kettlebells enable you to concoct cool combination exercises that deliver an unbelievable muscular and cardiovascular workout in a very short period time. Take this evil combo, courtesy of Comrade D. C. Maxwell:

Do the deck squat. When you are up, immediately switch your grip on the kettlebell and snatch it. Drop the bell, regrip again, and roll back in a deck squat. Enjoy!

More combo suggestions:

- One-arm swing + clean-and-press + snatch

- Clean-and- -press + overhead squat

- Overhead squat + military press

- Front squat + military press

- Front squat + military press + snatch

- Front squat + military press + overhead squat

- Turkish getup + one-legged military press

The number of reps on every part of the combo doesn't have to be the same. For instance, in the first combo, you might do 5 swings, 1 press, and 3 snatches. Be creative and realistic about your strength and weakness. You won't be able to press the bell nearly as many times as you can swing it.

Some combos may be done in one circuit; others can go on for a few rounds. If you get bored training with kettlebells, someone must have amputated your imagination.

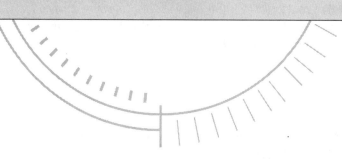

Just like yoga with the WINDMILL

Treat your kettlebell practice as yoga

According to famous yoga teacher B. K. S. Iyengar, the word yoga was derived from the Sanskrit root *yuj*, which means "to bind, join, attach and yoke, to direct one's attention on, to use and apply." Like yoga and unlike conventional resistance training, *From Russia with Tough Love* focuses on the mind, muscle, and breathing connection and despises mindless and endless repetition.

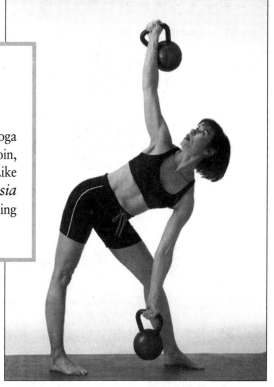

Russian yoga

RKC—The Russian answer to yoga?
From: Pietro
I've only finished my fourth KB workout and have found that it is much like yoga. Now before you scoff at this remark, I'm sure you, too, have noticed many similarities. In yoga, flexing of the rectal, abdominal, and various other locks and muscles is required—much like RKC'. Yoga uses "Ujayi" breathing to retain body heat, tension, and mindfulness—much like RKC'.

Yoga flows from one posture to another very smoothly with transition movements (Ashtanga yoga, anyway)—much like windmills, chest-opening windmills, side press and military presses can blend into each other. Also, yoga requires the utmost concentration and focus for it to be truly beneficial—much like RKC', where concentration and focus on tension and the weight are needed for progress in strength, muscular endurance, and to keep from dropping the damn weight on your head! One last thing: I feel so doggone energized and alive after RKC'—this time, much like yoga!

Side presses help with many asanas
From: Master Rinpoche
I can do side bends and triangle pose better than almost anyone in my Yoga class, and I am a rank beginner. I am pretty sure this is because I have flexible strength from doing the side-presses.

My wife says windmills are yoga with weights (n/m)
From: SteveFreides

Big fan of windmills!
From: Davidh
I just love doing windmills. I guess it's the slow bending, twisting stretching motion going down and the whole body contraction getting back up. It is very invigorating. Maybe it's the almost yoga like feel to it that is so stimulating. I always feel better after doing two or three sets.

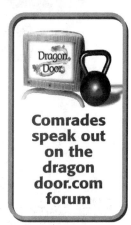

Comrades speak out on the dragon door.com forum

Windmill

The Art of Kettlebelling

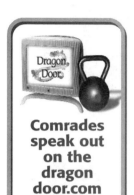

People of Dragon Door!
From: Barry1001
The KB marries strength, agility, balance, and technique. Primitive yet sophisticated. A minute to learn, a lifetime to master.

Re: PTP or KB?
From: drc__
About a month ago, I got the 16-kg model to see whether K-bells were all that

I'd heard. I was not disappointed. Great workouts, and it's fun. The K-bell is frequently compared to the dumbbell, but that comparison misses some points. In some ways, the K-bell is like a gymnastics apparatus—say, the horse or the high bar. It rewards skill but does not require an extraordinary skill, like the gymnast or Olympic lifter. The K-bell invites improvisation, even play.

Here's an unreal drill for a powerful and flexible waist, back, and hips. It looks a lot like yoga's Trikonasana, but it's not the same, so please pay attention to the differences.

Stand with your feet slightly wider than your shoulders, and pivot until your left foot points almost to the side and your right is at an approximately 30-degree angle. Stick the ridges of your hands into your hip creases, just the way you did when practicing the "Good Morning" stretch, and push so your weight shifts to your nearly straight back leg and your butt sticks out. Please note the incorrect position shown in the photo: the weight slipping to the front leg.

Good Form

Poor Form

• Stick the ridges of your hands into your hip creases, just the way you did when practicing the "Good Morning" stretch, and push so your weight shifts to your nearly straight back leg and your butt sticks out.

• Don't let your weight slip forward or your knees bow in.

Windmill

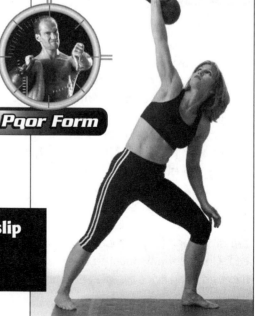

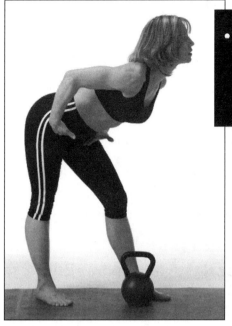

• **Stand with your feet slightly wider than your shoulders, and pivot until your left foot points almost to the side and your right is at an approximately 30-degree angle.**

And here's another example of an incorrect and dangerous foot position: the feet pointing in a direction other than specified (for example, forward) and the knees bowing in.

Rotate your torso, your chest wide open, so your arms reach out as wide apart as possible—your right toward the ceiling and your left toward the floor. It helps to let out a sigh of relief on the bottom to increase your range of motion. Look at your top hand.

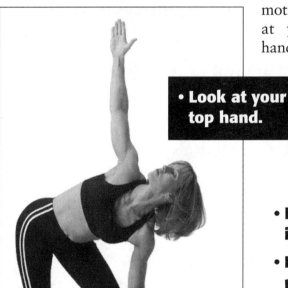

Poor Form

• **Don't let the knees bow in.**

• **Don't let the feet point forward.**

• **Look at your top hand.**

• **Let out a sigh of relief on the bottom to increase your range of motion.**

• **Feel for the kettlebell that has been parked by your ankle. Take it.**

• **Rotate your torso, your chest wide open, so your arms reach out as wide apart as possible—your right toward the ceiling and your left toward the floor.**

Windmill

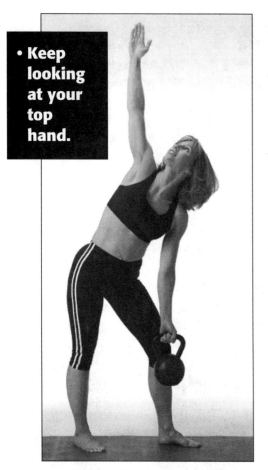

• Keep looking at your top hand.

Feel for the kettlebell that has been parked by your ankle. (You may have to lift it off a box if you aren't yet flexible enough to lift it off the ground.) Take it. Inhale, squeeze your right glute (extremely important!), and slowly come up, following the exact path of your descent. If you straighten out in some other fashion, you are likely to get hurt.

Keep driving with your glute, steady and powerful, until you end up in the position shown—your glute cramped and your hip assertively pushed forward.

Go down for another rep while carefully releasing your air. Naturally, work both sides.

- **Inhale, squeeze your right glute (extremely important!), and slowly come up, following the exact path of your descent.**

- **Keep driving with your glute, steady and powerful, until you lock out your hips.**

- **Go down for another rep while carefully releasing your air.**

- **Work both sides.**

Strengthen and harden, don't build

Few drills can touch the windmill when it comes to molding hard obliques. But beware of overdoing it on the volume; too many windmills could thicken your waist. As a rule of thumb, do no more than 12 repetitions per side per workout, preferably in multiple sets of low reps, such as 4x3, 3x4, and 5x2. Don't be afraid to go heavy; just don't do too many reps and avoid the pump.

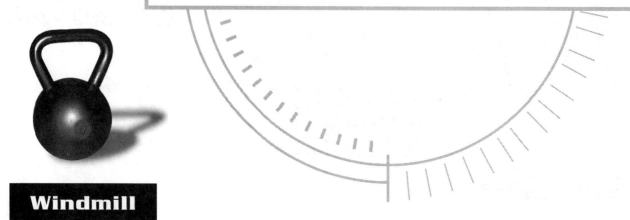

Windmill

Once you have mastered the windmill with the kettlebell held near the floor, advance to the windmill with the kettlebell held overhead.

Elevate a kettlebell safely overhead any way you like, and kick out your right hip to the side. As before, keep your right knee locked or nearly locked, and maintain as much weight as possible on your right leg throughout the stretch. The other knee may be bent; this is not the triangle pose from yoga, Comrade! Again, note the position of the feet.

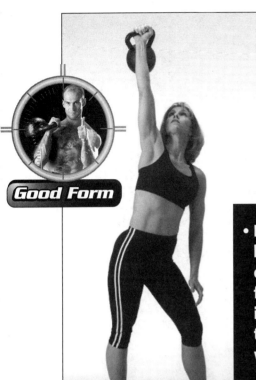

Good Form

• **Elevate a kettlebell safely overhead, and follow the instructions for the first type of windmill.**

• **Punch into the sky with a firm arm, using the same technique as that of the overhead squats.**

Punch to the sky with your firm arm, as during overhead squats. Note the bad arm and shoulder position in the photo: bent and weakly disconnected from the body.

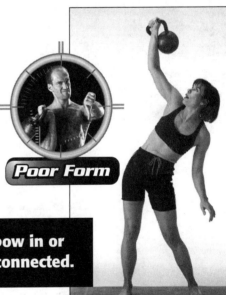

Poor Form

• **Don't let the knees bow in or the arm become disconnected.**

Keep your chest open and your eyes on the bell. Release some air, and fold forward—never backward!—and to the side.

• **Keep the arm solid and strong.**

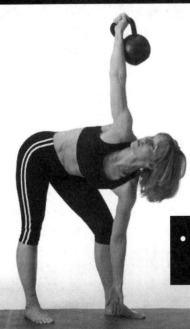

• **Go as deep as you can safely go.**

Windmill

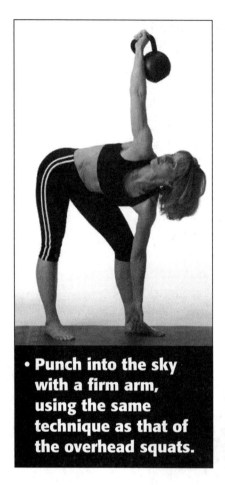

• **Punch into the sky with a firm arm, using the same technique as that of the overhead squats.**

This action is similar to jackknifing in the "Good Morning" stretch but is done more to the side than to the rear. If you are not yet flexible enough to go that deep, only go as deep as you safely can. You may set a stool or a yoga block of an appropriate height as a target to touch.

When you have reached the limit of your depth in good form, squeeze your glutes and slowly, without twisting, get up, following the "groove" you made on the way down. It helps to grip the ground with your toes.

• **Grip the ground with your toes, especially on the way up.**

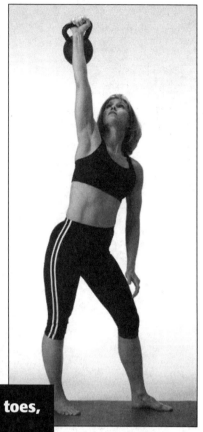

Comrades saying goodbye to their glass backs

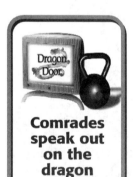

Comrades speak out on the dragon door.com forum

The revenge of the curse of the kettlebell
From: Barely Sane
Has anyone else found that bent/side presses and windmills have a restorative effect on the lower back? I managed to twang something while doing enthusiastic clean-and-jerks (with sloppy form). But one day later, since I can't seem to leave the KBs alone,

I returned to bent pressing, VERY strictly, and my low-back pain went bye-bye.

Re: Pavel KP?
From: drc__
When I first started using Pavel's methods (January of this year), I had my doubts about my ability to perform the movements. I had a history of various

back pains, some quite severe. I gave it a shot, nonetheless, and my back has not felt this good in over 20 years. PTP [Power to the People] and RKC' have been a blessing to me.

Snatches cure back pain!
From: Ari
A month ago, I took off some time from RKC' because my wrists were starting to hurt a bit from going overboard on the volume. After a few days off, my back just started to kill. I was dreading going back to the RKC' because of this back pain. But wouldn't you know it, with a few days of snatches under my belt, the back pain just melted away! Unbelievable. So many people have back pain just from inactivity and weakness. Wish some of my friends would wake up and get

Windmill

Once you get the basic windmill down pat, place your hand behind your back. Aim to lay your chest on your knee eventually.

The great Canadian strong man George Jowett colorfully describes the benefits of the hand-behind-the-back windmill: "You will find this exercise a dandy in more respects than one. Here is a peach for giving your entire back a workout in contraction and extension. The first time you practice it, you will feel a sensation upon your breast bone and in your shoulders akin to spreading apart." (Seems this awesome exercise used to be popular on this side of the pond, as well.)

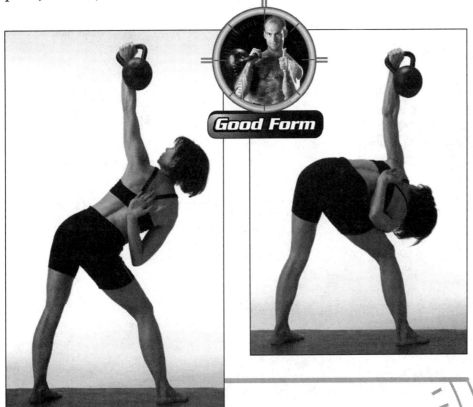

Good Form

Match your breath with the force

Matching the breath with the force is a very important power-generation concept from the martial arts. You must pressurize your abdomen for the exact duration of exertion. That's why we use different Power Breathing variations for different drills: hissing, grunting, holding a pressurized breath, keeping your abdomen pressurized but breathing shallow.

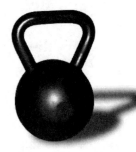

Windmill

Another advanced windmill variation calls for two kettlebells. Hold one overhead then get down to lift the other one from between your feet. Note how the hips punch through at the top. You may use kettlebells of different sizes; if you do, the smaller one goes to the top.

You will notice that the two-kettlebells windmill gives you a more intense contraction through a limited range of motion. It's wonderful for hard love handles and creating a stable spine. The hand-behind-the-back variation is an exercise in flexibility as much as strength.

> • **You may use kettlebells of different sizes; if you do, the smaller one goes to the top.**

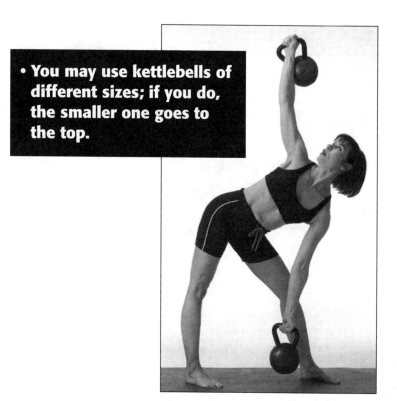
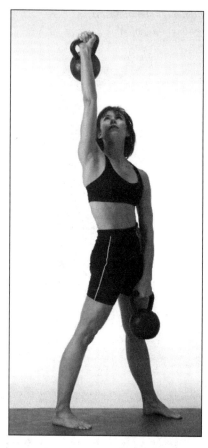

The bottoms-up press rocks!

Bottoms-up press
From: Scotty

I just wanted to encourage everyone to try the bottoms-up press if you haven't yet. I started with it a few weeks ago and had amazing results. After doing it for only a week, I switched back to normal presses and found that the "standard" military press was now much easier. I then went back to working hard on the bottoms-up press and continued to gain. The only problem is that my KB is now too light!

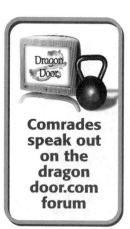

Comrades speak out on the dragon door.com forum

Windmill

Forge iron wrists and grip and firm up your waist with the BOTTOMS-UP CLEAN-AND-PRESS

The following deceptively simple kettlebell exercise —a clean or clean-and-press but done upside down—works wonders on your grip and wrists as well as your waist.

You will quickly realize that unless you explosively grip the kettlebell's handle just at the right moment and brace and pressurize your abdomen (grunt!) at the same time, you won't stand a chance. The kettlebell will flop down. Consider getting a spotter.

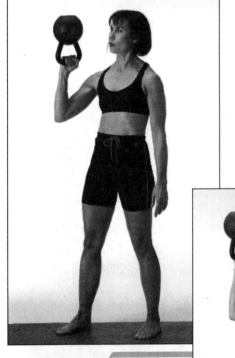

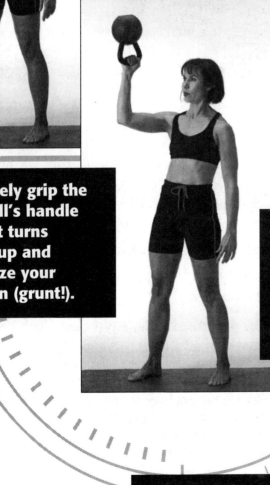

• Explosively grip the kettlebell's handle just as it turns bottom up and pressurize your abdomen (grunt!).

• If the kettlebell flops down. Consider getting a spotter.

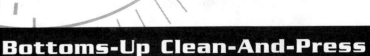

Bottoms-Up Clean-And-Press

Start by practicing cleans only in sets of 3 to 5 reps. Aim for a total synchronization of your breath and the force.

Once you can consistently freeze the KB in your hand with its bottom up (the balance is achieved by squeezing the handle, not by moving nonstop, trying to catch up with the falling bell!), you may try the press, also for very low reps. Maintain total body tension, or suffer total failure! Try applying the tension skills you have learned to other kettlebell drills. You will also be pleasantly surprised that the bottoms-up clean-and-press improves your striking power in martial arts, tennis, golf, and more.

Get an even harder stomach and tie you upper and lower body into a strong unit with the ROLLING SITUP

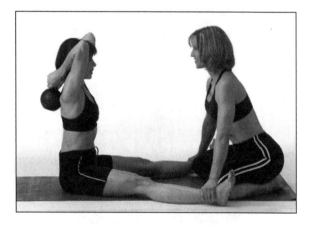

If your back and stomach are strong and healthy, then try the following remarkable old kettlebell favorite: the rolling situp. It will feel great and work wonders for you.

Sit on the floor with your legs straight in front of you, your feet wider than your shoulders. Have your training partner firmly hold your ankles down. Safely get the kettlebell in the position behind your upper back. You can also first practice the rolling situp without any weight at all.

- **Sit on the floor with your legs straight in front of you, your feet wider than your shoulders.**
- **Have your training partner firmly hold your ankles down.**
- **Safely get the kettlebell in the position behind your upper back.**
- **Take a breath, firm up your right glute, tuck in your tail, brace your abs, and simultaneously roll slowly a little to the right and back.**
- **Great glute tension is vital for protecting your lower back.**

Rolling Situp

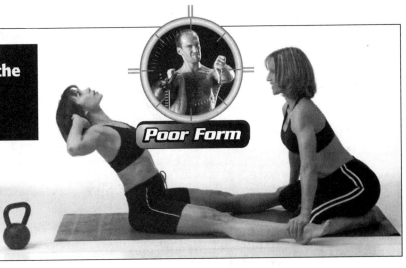

• You can also first practice the rolling situp without any weight at all

• Your spine can be straight or rounded but not arched!

Poor Form

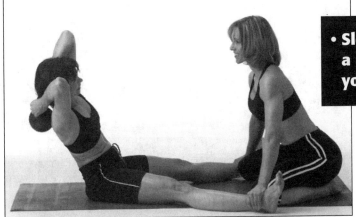

• Slowly roll, making a small circle with your torso

Take a breath, firm up your right glute, tuck in your tail, brace your abs, and simultaneously roll slowly a little to the right and back. Your spine can be straight or rounded but not arched!

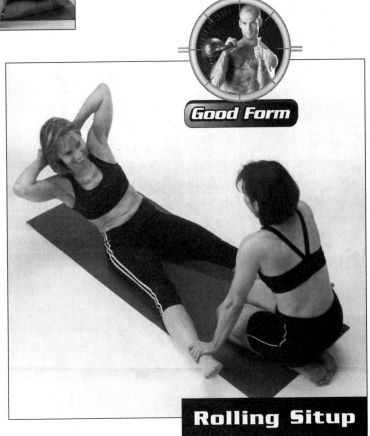

Good Form

Rolling Situp

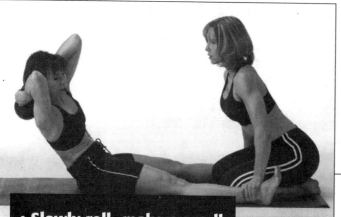

Slowly roll, making a small circle with your torso. Take shallow breaths in order to keep your waist tight. Come back to the center, then tense your left cheek, and then roll the other way. Great glute tension is vital for protecting your lower back.

• **Slowly roll—make a small circle with your torso.**

Good Form

• **Come back to the center, then tense your left cheek, and roll the other way.**

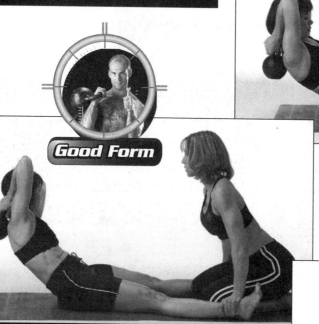

• **Finally, roll forward and release your air in a sigh of relief to stretch your hamstrings and back.**

• **Now circle the other way.**

• **If you can do it safely, go lower.**

• **Take shallow breaths in order to keep your waist tight.**

Rolling Situp

Finally, roll forward and release your air in a sigh of relief. Your hamstrings and back will feel pleasantly stretched.

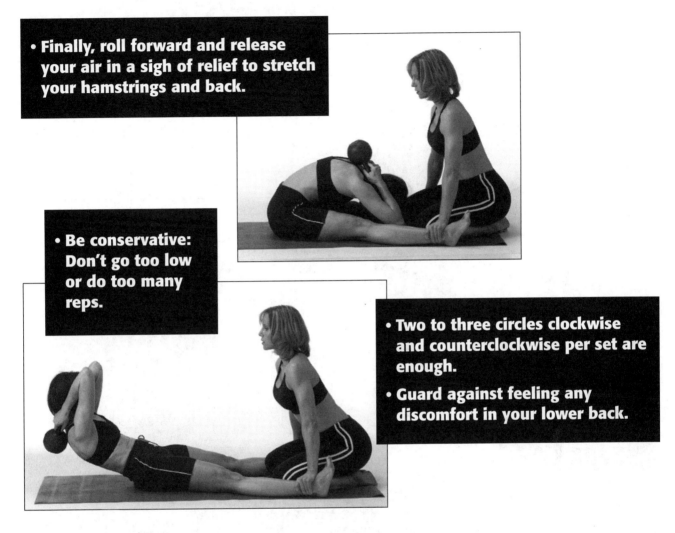

- **Finally, roll forward and release your air in a sigh of relief to stretch your hamstrings and back.**

- **Be conservative: Don't go too low or do too many reps.**

- **Two to three circles clockwise and counterclockwise per set are enough.**
- **Guard against feeling any discomfort in your lower back.**

Now circle the other way. If you can do it safely, go lower.

Be conservative! Don't go too low or do too many reps. Two to three circles clockwise and counterclockwise per set are enough. Your back will thank you for it.

Recall this feeling of the upper- and lower-body unity when you do other exercises.

Rolling Situp

Cut up your legs and burn calories with the DRAGON WALK

My friend and publisher, John Du Cane, taught me this Chi Kung exercise, the dragon walk, as an evil alternative to the lunge. Do yourself a favor and start without extra weights. Then progress to holding a kettlebell in front of you and finally to two K-bells held as shown.

• **Your ankles will cross, but your knees must always track your feet.**

• **Stay upright throughout**

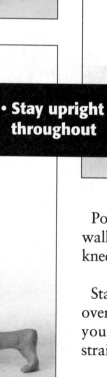

Points to observe when you are dragon walking: Your ankles will cross, but your knees should always track your feet.

Stay upright throughout. If you fold over, squeezing your glutes and pushing your hips forward will help you straighten out.

Dragon Walk

Your knee should come down to within an inch of the ground but not actually touch it. This isn't easy, so don't attempt the dragon walk until your leg strength is way above average.

Also, note that your knee should end up exactly outside your leading ankle. You will have to experiment with the length of your step to get it right.

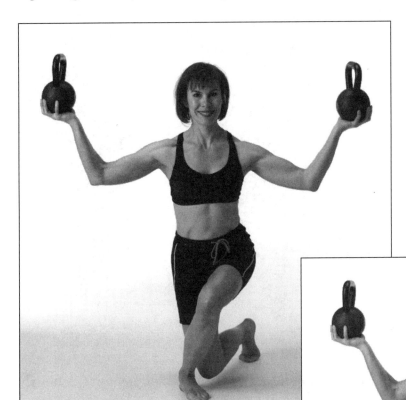

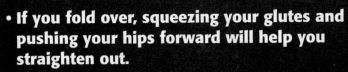

- **If you fold over, squeezing your glutes and pushing your hips forward will help you straighten out.**
- **Your knee should come down to within an inch of the ground but not actually touch it.**

- **Your knee should end up exactly outside your leading ankle; experiment with the length of your step to get it right.**

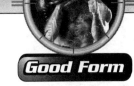

Good Form

Dragon Walk

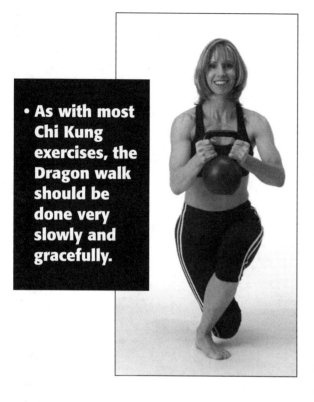

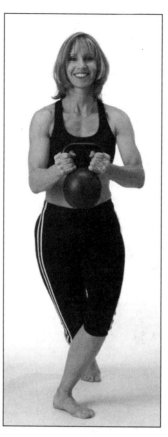

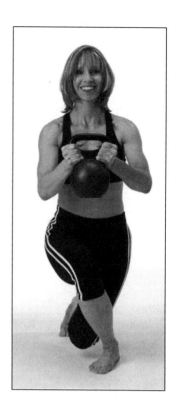

• As with most Chi Kung exercises, the Dragon walk should be done very slowly and gracefully.

Although John Du Cane can dragon walk for an hour straight, it's definitely no walk in the park for mere mortals. Enjoy the pain!

If you like the dragon walk

Do yourself a favor and check out the John Du Cane's videotape set, *The Five Animal Frolics*. You will find what you want to know about John's awesome program in the end of this book. Chi Kung has so much to offer to your well-being. Quoting John himself, "Manage stress, reduce pain, restore energy, and heal yourself with the highly effective and pleasurable methods of Chinese Qigong."

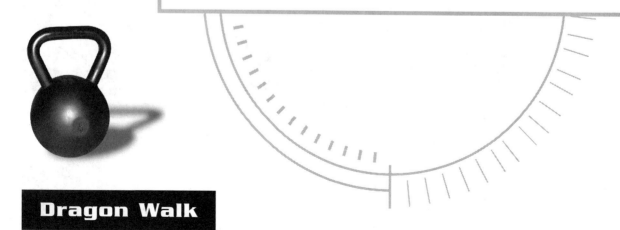

Dragon Walk

The infinity of kettlebell drills

You've probably realized by now that you can use your kettlebells in way more exercises than are listed in this book. You can use kettlebells to do everything you can do with dumbbells—only better—plus much more (such as the bottoms-up clean-and-press). I don't want to waste your time going over the obvious lunges and curls, and you should have the knowledge at this point to invent plenty of drills on your own. IPO whole paragraph

If you get bitten by the curiosity bug, consider the following additional kettlebell resources:

- *The Russian Kettlebell Challenge: Xtreme Fitness for Hard Living Comrades* [book], **by yours truly**
  This book will teach you a few new tricks and routines plus the history of kettlebells and some more things. While written with men in mind, it works just as well for women. (Just ignore the exhaustive variations of upper-body drills; you know better to focus on your "rear-wheel drive.")

- *The Russian Kettlebell Challenge: Xtreme Fitness for Hard Living Comrades* [video], **by yours truly**
  The video will demonstrate the basics you know plus some that you don't, such as jerks and under-the-leg passes. Some extreme drills, such as bent presses, are shown, too.

- *Steve Maxwell's Cruel and Unusual Kettlebell Exercises for Real Men* [video]
  Don't be put off by the macho title of this tape. At the end, Steve's wife, D. C., comes in, puts a hurt on him, and sets the record straight: It's for real women, too. If you happen to be in Philadelphia, stop by at the Maxwells' studio, Maxercise, for a great kettlebell plus personal workout or a KB class. The number is (215) 928-1374.

- **Certified Russian Kettlebell Challenge (RKC) instructors**
  Our instructors are top notch. You may want to work with a trainer full time or just buy a few sessions to get into the groove or to learn some new moves. Contact information for instructors is provided at dragondoor.com.

- **Certified Russian Kettlebell Challenge (RKC) instructor course**
  You can register for this intense, one-of-a-kind workshop at dragondoor.com.

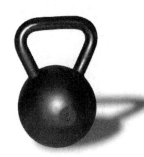

• **Dragondoor.com forum**
We host what we believe is the classiest training discussion site on the Internet. Learn a lot about kettlebells and other fitness topics.

• **Dragondoor.com free articles**
A number of free quality articles are posted on the site, many of them dedicated to kettlebell training.

• *Pavel's Power To The People! E-Newsletter*
Sign up for my free fitness e-newsletter on the dragondoor.com home page.

From Russia with Tough Love
Freestyle Kettlebell Training

One of the great advantages of kettlebell training is its tremendous versatility. Once you have spent a couple of months mastering the drills and learning to listen to your body, you will be ready for freestyle kettlebelling.

1. Use your good judgment, and listen to your body.

In a book or in person, I cannot possibly cover all the contingencies of kettlebell or any other type of fitness training. "Don't drop your kettlebell on your head; you could get killed! " Duh!

If a student at the RKC instructor certification course does something unsafe, I immediately punish him or her with a set of pushups. The infractions vary Jumping to a heavier KB prematurely. Picking up a kettlebell improperly. Wearing shoes that slide on a given surface. Standing too close to another student when performing dynamic overhead drills. Trying to save a bad lift when getting the hell out of the way and dropping the bell like a hot potato was the right thing to do.

With corporal punishment, I cultivate common sense, and I'm pleased to say that it works. Unless you attend an RKC instructor certification course, you won't have the dubious pleasure of me barking at you for doing something stupid. So, *please use your brain!* No matter what the book, the tape, or your trainer says, if something doesn't feel right, don't do it.

If a routine specifies 3 sets to the limit and you don't feel that great, do fewer sets or less reps. If your knee aches, see a doctor instead of doing squats. If you aren't limber enough to do the windmill, don't do it until you develop the flexibility or do it but barely go down an inch or so. If you feel stiff and rundown all the time and have a hard time sleeping, cut back on your training, no matter what the schedule says.

If, on the other hand, you breeze through the outlined workouts, crank it up and do more. Your body should feel right. Period.

Obvious as it is, that is the first commandment of kettlebell training and any physical activity, for that matter.

2. Train as often as possible while being as fresh as possible.

Russian researchers discovered that fragmentation of the training volume into smaller units is very effective for promoting strength adaptation, especially in the nervous system. (Read *without building muscle mass*.) In other words, 1 set 6 days a week is superior to 2 sets 3 times a week. Professor Vladimir Zatsiorsky summed up effective strength building as *training as often as possible while being as fresh as possible*.

Russian yoga

D. C.'s comments on Pavel's workout at the Arnold [Schwarzenegger's Fitness Expo]

From: D. C. Maxwell

This is D. C., Steve's wife. I had the unique pleasure (I think) of having Pavel himself put me through some KB paces at the Arnold show in Ohio this past weekend. I had made the request for the workout the previous evening at dinner, and Pavel had accepted. Not being a workout masochist, I tried to make sure he knew that this was not a challenge, but to no avail. Right in front of the Dragon Door booth, he put me through a workout that almost made me bleed from the eyeballs. I'm just a 125-pound woman who's very normal (i.e., no threat to either the fitness babes or the muscle women who populated the show). Pavel drilled me through snatches, shoulder presses, more snatches, and turkish getups with the 36-pounder. He made me do one-legged deadlifts with the 72-pounder. More snatches with the 36-pounder but holding a heavier KB with my other hand. It's largely a blur, but somewhere during this workout, a sympathetic crowd had gathered. As he topped off my workout with 50 rockups ("Did I say stop?") and a couple of sets on the new Ab Pavelizer, I kept the images of my children in my mind to retain the will to live. Afterward, I crawled over to Ori Hofmekler for a dose of Warrior's Milk and then back to my hotel room for a nap.

Although I am married to one of the country's premier KB trainers, it was great to have the Pavel experience. Thanks, Pavel.

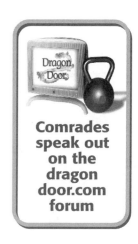

Comrades speak out on the dragon door.com forum

Try to train daily, if you can. Better yet, chop up your daily workload into multiple mini-sessions. Motor-learning Comrades know that while the total number of trials is important, the frequency of practice is even more critical. Naturally, if all you can find is 30 minutes twice a week, it's better than nothing. Much better.

Don't freak out about training the same movement or the same body part for many days in a row. That's standard operating procedure among Russian athletes. In fact, the Russian National Powerlifting Team benches up to 8 times a week.

Let me give you another reason to maximize your training frequency: Doing even 1 set of a kettlebell exercise will spike your metabolism and activate the fat-burning machinery. Just grabbing your kettlebell here and there throughout the day for a quick set or two will work magic on your body.

3. Cycle

Varying the training load from day to day will help you make quicker progress, according to Russian scientists, such as former weightlifting world champion Professor Arkady Vorobyev.

Wave the following parameters up and down, though not necessarily all at once:

The length of the workout—This is an indirect way to manipulate the training load. Workouts between 1 and 45 minutes are fine.

Relative intensity Relative intensity refers to how close you come to your limit or repetition maximum (RM). For instance, test your limit in the one-arm snatch (stop 1 rep before failure), but do only two-thirds of the reps you could normally do with the pedal to the metal on the deck squat (65% relative intensity).

Sets—Generally, you should do between 1 and 5 sets per drill, unless you employ interval or ladder training (see below). Eventually, you may be doing more. Listen to your body, and use your head.

Repetitions—The important thing is to stop before your form starts deteriorating; otherwise, you have carte blanche to do as many reps as you can handle—1 to 100 plus.

Multiple sets of low reps are recommended for exercises that require a lot of coordination, especially slow lifts such as the military press. Say, you aim for a high volume—high total reps—in the overhead squat. Do 1 to 5 reps with the bell in one hand, and then switch hands. If you keep switching back and forth in this fashion, with or without rest, your smaller and weaker shoulders will be able to keep up with your powerful legs.

And forget the myth that "Low reps are for bulking, and high reps are for toning." The reality is that "High calories are for bulking, and low calories are for toning."

Rest periods between sets—*High motor density*, or the amount of work performed per unit of time, is an important component of effective endurance training and fat loss. But beware of compressing your rest intervals so much that your technique goes south.

"Listen to your body" is the best advice you can get regarding optimal rest. And don't passively hang around; keep moving (walking around or jogging in place) to help your heart.

Tempo—Russian researcher S. Lelikov (1975) discovered that strength programs that vary the exercise tempo are much more effective than those that do not. So periodically speed up or slow down your movement to get away from a comfortable pace. For example, snatch either at the limit of your explosiveness or at a near stall. When pressing, lower the kettlebell fast but lift it slow or vice versa . Training to different-paced music is another option.

Exercise order—It's up to you to shuffle things up. A couple of guidelines, though:

- Be sure to practice the moves that require a lot of precision, such as windmills, when you are fresh.

- Figure out how to arrange your drills in a way that will have the minimal negative effect on your performance. For instance, after doing military presses and snatches, your shoulders will be shot. Give your shoulders a break by doing something like the deck squat or the one-legged deadlift before going back to more exercises involving the shoulders, like the front squat.

- Alternate between harder and easier (for you) exercises and/or sets. For example, do a set of 5 reps in the difficult military press and then 10 reps in the relatively easy two-arm swing.

- If you have a weakness you would like to address, use the time-tested Russian practice of starting and finishing your workout with the same exercise.

Although circuit training should not be your only choice, it works well in a *From Russia with Tough Love* workout. Going from one exercise to another enables the trainee to handle a greater volume of training, thanks to the phenomenon of *fatigue specificity*. A Comrade's ability to repeat the drill he or she has just performed recovers a lot more slowly than his or her ability to do other exercises, even when the same muscle groups are involved. In other words, a change of activity is a form of rest. Circuit training doesn't mean you have to rush from one drill to another; you may rest a bit in between, which is so-called interval circuit training.

Number exercises— Shifting between smorgasbord routines that contain one or two exercise workouts is good for the body and the head.

If you want to add *Bullet-Proof Abs, Power to the People!* or some other exercise to your kettlebell regimen, plug your deadlifts and other favorite moves into your kettlebell sessions and make them play by the rules outlined here.

Weight—The beauty of the *From Russia with Tough Love* workout is that you don't need a ton of dumbbells of different sizes or an expensive set of adjustable ones. Kettlebell workouts are designed to provide great variety and deliver a powerful training effect using only one or two sizes of KBs. But once you do get strong enough to use a heavier kettlebell, you will have made a great and easy choice of workout design. Just alternate the bells from workout to workout; you will be forced to cycle the variables we have discussed, and you will find it's easy on your head.

The no-hassle workout

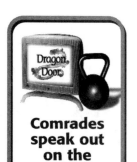

Comrades speak out on the dragon door.com forum

Smart decision
From: ScotPower

I used to get all mentally tied up figuring out when I was going to squat, bench, deadlift, etc.; eat and sleep for "max gains"; and all that. Maybe I'm just a little older now. I just grab the K-bells whenever I feel like it and do it. Barefoot, just me in my boxer shorts.

So much time left for all the other stuff...

Why KBs rock, Part XIV
From: Rob Lawrence

I've decided my favorite thing about KBs is that you don't have to load and unload a bar! That's always my least favorite part of a workout. Although I love doing deads, I hate setting up the bar and wasting time. It makes it easy to lose focus, particularly when you're training for wiry strength and don't want to let an eon go by between sets. I've tried substituting barbell versions for KB lifts in my routine for variety, but I've decided the variety is not worth the time lapse. I prefer to attack the iron and keep working. Call me impatient, if you will.

From: Matthias

I totally agree. I spend much more time actually working out now instead of trying to decide if I'm going to do straight sets or pyramids or drop sets or whatever. And it's nice not to have to constantly clean out and reorganize the garage to make room for a 7-foot bar. Every time I walk into my living room, there's my double (and my wife's half), just waiting there, ready for action.

Another way to cycle your workouts

"For a faster rate of improvement and better recuperation in a weekly cycle it makes sense to vary your loads," write Russian specialists A. Burkov and V. Nikityuk. "For that reason one ought to increase the volume in one of the weekly workouts (by approximately 10%) in each set and perform the last set of each exercise to the limit and with maximal speed."

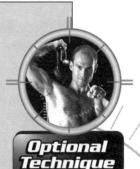

Two great alternatives to straight sets

Interval training is very productive. Say, you can do 50 box squats if you go all out. But instead, you do 6 sets of 10 with 10-second rest breaks in between. Or you do 10 sets of 10 with 30 seconds of rest. You get the idea.

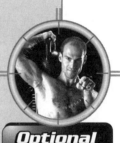

The ladder is a Russian Special Forces favorite. Do 1 rep and set the weight down. Rest for as long as it would take another Comrade to do what you just did. Then do 2 reps. Then 3. And so on. When things get really ugly, start all over at 1 or move on to the next exercise. You can come back for more later.

As an option, you may terminate the ladder at an earlier chosen rep count instead of fighting till the bitter end. With very high-rep drills, such as swings, you may take larger steps—for instance, 5-10-15 reps.

Ladder success stories abound on the dragondoor.com training forum.

Overtraining:
Take a lemon and make lemonade

Soviet coaches realized that the waiting for complete recovery between workouts could take an athlete only so far. Indeed, *controlled overtraining*—known in the United States as *overreaching*—followed by a tapering off, leads to gains far superior to those possible with total-recovery training.

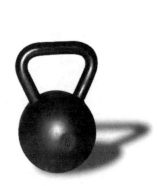

Although the Russians employ some very sophisticated controlled-overtraining models, this doesn't have to be rocket science. Once you get in a good shape, you can article he has posted on dragondoor.com. Rogers works his whole body for 2 or 3 days in a row. Then he either takes a day or two off or tapers with very easy active-recovery training. Push, back off, push, back off . . .

If you like your training cycle to fit nicely into the week, try training Monday through Thursday and then taking Friday through Sunday off. Whatever plan you choose, it's essential that you listen to your body. Overreaching is a powerful tool, but if abused, it can lead to overuse injuries and systemic problems. As explained by former world weightlifting champion Professor Arkady Vorobyev, "Constant training on the background of incomplete restoration can have dangerous consequences . . . [such as] chronic fatigue and overtraining. Therefore the organism needs a chance to recover completely." So use your head!

If you're a beginner, don't try to overtrain and only use this model if you accidentally stumble into it. Overreaching for 1 week every month is more than adequate for an experience trainee. You will experience great fitness gains; surprisingly, most of the improvement will likely take place during the first week of going back to conventional full-recovery training.

I urge you not to misinterpret this observation as touting the superiority of full-recovery training. This is a delayed adaptation made possible by earlier overreaching. Vorobyev explains that incomplete restoration training stimulates the recovery ability; your body literally has to learn how to recoup faster or else! To give you an analogy, say you signed up to work as a logger and went home very sore after your first day of work. If you persisted and kept logging day after day, through soreness and fatigue, your body would eventually adapt and have no problem handling the daily grind. On the other hand, if you were allowed to work only when you had totally recovered (an unlikely option, for sure), you would work twice a week at the most and always recover slowly and painfully. (Sound familiar?)

By taxing your recovery ability through intense daily training, you will be building up your adaptation reserves. When you finally go back to pumping up each muscle every 3 to 5 days, your muscles will fill out like never before! As a Lithuanian saying goes, "A river with a dam has more power."

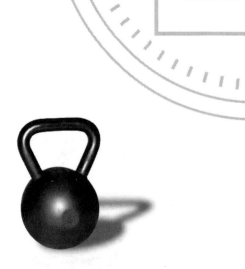

The Party says: "Kettlebells rule!"

OH, yeah—best training tool, ever
From: CarolynLibrarian

Those "cute little cannonballs," as one troll once put, it are—technically speaking—da bomb. I've made incredible strength and endurance gains in just a few weeks.

LOL: I can just see "Turnip Boy" getting all apoplectic over this and then trying desperately hard to outdo you. Failing miserably. BUT HE'S GOT THE GUNS, MANNNNNNN!!!!! What good are 20-inch arms if they're 70% water?

Kettlebells may not make me strong enough to win a strongwoman competition, but they are by far the best conditioning tool I've ever seen, bar none. And a helluva a way to build functional strength overall.

All this, in only a few minutes a day. Having actual fun. Amazing.

My plan for world domination is right on schedule.
Re: KB update
From: Lemon

Well, my girlfriend noticed a distinct change for the better in my build and appearance after about 3 weeks of K-bells, and it took about 3 more before anyone else made a comment about it (seeing me in street clothes).

Com. Pavel: as requested, "How I Have Changed With a Year of RKC"
From: JasonC

1) I'm one healthy comrade, and everybody I know envies my energy. This is NOT the old me.

2) I can be as lean as I want to be. Training with KBs, I can eat anything I please and not balloon. In the springtime, to lean out some, I just eat fewer carbs, and I get nice and sleek.

3) I have the "look of power…"

4) Visible abs.

5) Endurance. One of the happiest days of my athletic life was when I introduced a former Army medevac pilot to KB snatches. He watched me crank out 60-some 1-pood snatches per arm and said, "Hell, I know a lot of Rangers who couldn't keep up." Gotta love that…

Re: My wife is thinking about trying Kettlebells
From: Doughboy

She watched me working out with my KB when I first got it and she just kind of shook her head. I must have looked pretty goofy yanking that chunk of iron around.

Last night was when she first got interested. She noticed that in only a week of training with my KB I was getting thinner and more buff (which in my case is open to interpretation, but that's another story). I think I will start her on swings with the light DB. She will come over to the dark side soon enough.

Then I get to buy all the KB's I want.

Re: Kettlebell testimonies
From: Lemon

I did get a neat comment from an ex-girlfriend (we broke up and she married someone else, but we stayed on good terms) who saw me for the first time in a year, a year I spent working fairly hard on the K-bells:

"My God, what have you been DOING? You're like a ROCK. It's kind of SCARY!"

I am actually bigger, stronger, quicker, more athletic, and more muscular now, at 45, than I was at 32 when I was killing myself with 20-rep squats.

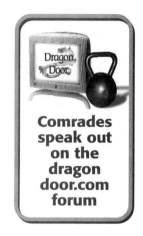

Comrades speak out on the dragon door.com forum

JOIN THE PARTY
www.dragondoor.com

The Party says: "Kettlebells rule!" (continued)

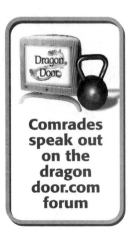

Comrades speak out on the dragon door.com forum

PARTY MEMBER
www.dragondoor.com

Re: Kettlebell testimonies
From: Barry1000

Excellent plan! I have been using the KB's for about 6 months. I have lost fat and gained muscle, and my energy level is fantastic. I have seen benefits in both running and in tennis; nothing replaces sport-specific training, but KB training seems to provide strength, endurance, and flexibility benefits that translate to better performance in a lot of activities. I feel like I am in better condition than I have been for 15 to 20 years.

Re: Kettlebell testimonies
From: BigNate

I'll put in my 2 cents, as well. You're very lucky to find KB's at your age. I started using them when I was 23 (I'm 24 now), and I wish I would have found them sooner. With KB's, I saw a drastic increase in my endurance for my grappling, the musculature of my whole body is harder, and cosmetically, I got development in my biceps that I was never able to get before KB's. Most importantly, I feel great and I get great satisfaction from the hard work required to get a good KB workout. KB's have helped me get my mind straight and be more focused in my training. Oh, I almost forgot: They improved my golf game, as well. I'm longer off the tee, and I feel I have more control over my entire swing. Good luck with them! You won't regret the purchase.

Re: Kettlebell testimonies
From: JohnnyK

Definitely get them. Everything you have read is true. No matter what I did to get more definition in my muscles, I couldn't do it. But with the KBs, I can see veins in my arms, freaky deltoid development; I can't even tell you what happened to my lats, and my legs are leaner and more powerful.

KB's make your muscles denser and harder. All in all, you are very lucky to have come across this information when you did—in fact, we are all lucky. Most of us wish we could have found it sooner!

I've added RKC explosive drills to my regimen with great success
From: Master Rinpoche

The bodyfat is melting off while my muscles seem to be getting "denser."

Someone I work with came up to me the other day and said, "You're getting in better shape right before my eyes."

Really—the results are so amazing, it's immensely motivating.

After 1 month
From: Steel

I have been using RKC' for about 1 month now. I have noted that my wind is better, and my forearm, delts, and back feel muuuuuuuch tighter. I enjoy doing the kettlebell workout and plan to use Comrade Pavel's training methods exclusively.

Testimonial on effects of KB's—longish
From: MarkWT

I know I'm mainly preaching to the choir here, but I wanted to share some of my results after using my new 1-pood KB for the past month. A month ago, I could only do 1 pullup. I'm a bit embarrassed to have to admit that here, but there you go. Today, having not tried to do any pullups for the past month, I did 3! Again, no great shakes around here, but a 300% improvement for me. A few minutes later, I did 3 again just to prove to myself that it wasn't a fluke. A few minutes later, I did 2. I might have been able to crank out another, but I didn't want to go to failure on it. I followed up with 3 dips—again, something I haven't been able to do before. I decided to try deadlifting. I'd only done it once in the past month and put 245 pounds on the bar—20 pounds heavier than I've ever done with the Olympic bar. I got it up! I did a set of 5 at that weight and finished with a 1x5 at 215 pounds. The lighter weight almost felt like it floated up.

Got my kb today!
BOINGGGGGGGGGGGG!!!!!!!!!!!!!!!
From: nikko

Are you kidding me? For any of you hem-hawing about getting a KB, quit wasting your time and just get it. Amazing workout. I can't wait till tomorrow.

What fun! I'm sold. Thanks for listening.
Mark

Re: Kettlebell testimonies
From: tylerhasselhoff
Since I started kettlebell training, I have become much more strong and muscular. I have gained about 8 pounds and lost some fat. My poundage in the deadlift has more than doubled, and my rep count in pullups has almost doubled.

Re: Kettlebell testimonies
From: Mongo
Lets see . . .
Gained 80 pounds on my deadlift.
Lost about 10 pounds of fat.
Great ab and back development.
Increased endurance in my martial arts.
Faster than going to the gym.

Re: Carolyn, welcome!!!!!!
From: tonya1980
WELCOME! It's great to hear your enthusiasm and motivation to get started with a new practice! You've discovered a gold mine. The main thing to remember is to pace yourself, use common sense, and it'll be a blast!!
Again, WELCOME!
Tonya
~Never, never underestimate the power of a woman lifting kettlebells!~

'Resistance is futile. You will be assimilated.'

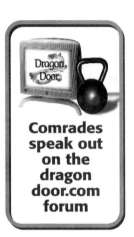

Comrades speak out on the dragon door.com forum

KB addiction and feeling of guilt!!!!!!!!!
From: Vaughan

I finally took a day off today 'cause I had an exam tonight, and I feel horribly guilty for taking the day off. I've developed an addiction to KB training. Not that it's a bad addiction to have, but I feel bad for not using it today—ike I've abandoned her or something (hahahaha). Hope my girlfriend doesn't read this!

Does anybody else have this addiction and feeling of guilt, or am I just messed up?

Pavel - A question about Smolov and KBs.....
From: exrecondoc

Pavel, I don't know if you put cocaine in the handles or something, but I can't keep my hands off my KB…

The fun has begun !
From: mead maker

This is without a doubt, the best, most addictive workout toy I've ever bought.

Re: KBs vs. spinning
From: GarrettPT

I gotta run. I hear my K-bells growling! Live long and strong.

Kettlebell control laws
From: MattZ

Forget gun control. With the army of mutants that Pavel has created, Congress may be looking to pass kettlebell control laws!

"They can have my kettlebell when they pry it from my cold, dead hand!"

I had a dream about swinging a kettlebell last night
From: dogchild

I've never done this in real life (yet), but it's becoming increasingly obvious that I will, one day, soon.

Count me among the seriously afflicted!

I love it, too! It's affecting my mind now!
From: Master Rinpoche

OK. So now I'm addicted to the KB exercises. Now I can't wait to get back into the gym. What the heck is wrong with me?

I think Pavel is using secret communist mind powers. I've said too much!

"The P-word today is performance, not *pink*."

This quote belongs to Anne Flannery, manager of women's athletics at Spalding. It's a scientific fact that looking at something pink even for a short period of time decreases one's

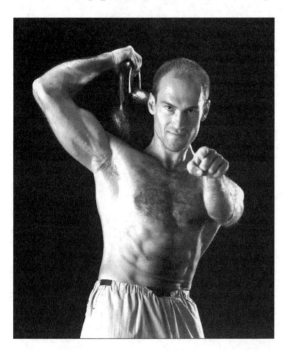

muscular strength. Clearly, the women's fitness movement has taken a wrong turn for the soft side.

Feminine does not equal **sissy**. Dispose of your pink Barbie weights. Say no to pink. See red!

Power to you!

Comrade Pavel

About the Author

Pavel

Pavel Tsatsouline, Master of Sports, was voted *Rolling Stone's* 'Hot Trainer' of the year in 2001. 'The Evil Russian' is the author of a number of best selling fitness books including *Relax into Stretch* and *Power to the People!* He is a contributing editor for Muscle Media magazine.

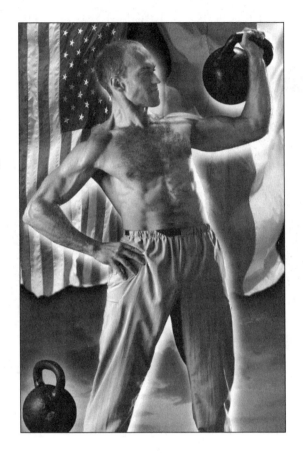

A former Soviet Special Forces instructor, Pavel was nationally ranked in the Russian ethnic sport of kettlebell lifting and holds a Soviet Physical Culture Institute degree in physiology and coaching. Tsatsouline teaches his '*low tech/high concept*' fitness approach to US military and law enforcement agencies and conducts national kettlebell instructor certification courses. Pavel has been interviewed by CNN Headline News, the Fox News Channel, USA Today, Associated Press, and EXTRA TV.

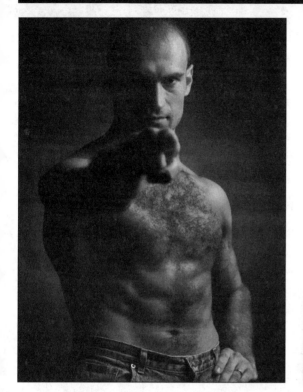

AMAZING NEWS:

Now You Can Carry a Whole Gym in One Hand—and Get a Fabulous,

TOTAL WORKOUT

Right in Your Own Living Room

- **Get picture-perfect slender**
- **Get lean, lean muscle tone**
- **Get way-faster fat loss**
- **Get firmer hips, thighs and butt**
- **Get into the slimmest, coolest, slinkiest clothes**
- **Get looked at twice—and then some**
- **Get the bust line you deserve and want**
- **Get a tremendous aerobic workout in half the time you used to take**

Each Russian Kettlebell is manufactured exclusively by Dragon Door Publications. The new kettlebells have a steel handle and a steel core surrounded by a rubber ball. These kettlebells are designed to last a lifetime—and beyond.

Special warning: Treat your kettlebell lifting with the utmost care, precision and respect. Watch Pavel's kettlebell video many, many times for perfect form and correct execution. If possible, sign up for one of Pavel's

upcoming Russian Kettlebell Challenge workshops.

Lift at your own discretion! We are not responsible for you boinking yourself on the head, dropping it on your feet or any other politically-incorrect action. Stick to the Party line, Comrade!

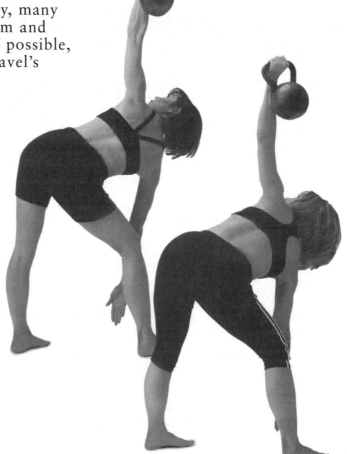

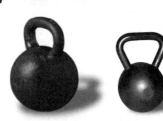

MANUFACTURED IN AMERICA

RUSSIAN KETTLEBELLS

SIZES DESIGNED FOR WOMEN

#	Size	Price	S/H
#P10D	4kg (approx. 9 lb)	$89.95	S/H: $10.00
#P10E	8kg (approx. 18 lb)	$99.95	S/H: $14.00

Until further notice, these new kettlebells are not available as a set.

CLASSIC KETTLEBELLS

#	Size	Price	S/H
#P10G	12kg (approx. 26lb)	$82.95	S/H: $20.00
#P10A	16kg (approx. 35lb)	$89.95	S/H: $24.00
#P10B	24kg (approx. 53lb)	$109.95	S/H: $32.00
#P10C	32kg (approx. 70lb)	$139.95	S/H: $39.00

NEW! 40kg SIZE—HEAVY METAL!

#	Size	Price	S/H
#P10F	40kg (approx. 88lb)	$179.95	S/H: $52.00

SAVE! ORDER A SET OF CLASSIC KETTLEBELLS AND SAVE $17.00!

#	Description	Price	S/H
#SP10	Set, one of A, B & C—16, 24 & 32kg. (Save $17.00)	$322.85	S/H: $95.00

The Russian Kettlebells are only available to customers resident in the U.S. mainland. Normal shipping charges do not apply. No rush orders on kettlebells.

"Download this tape into your eager cells and watch in stunned disbelief as your body reconstitutes itself, almost overnight"

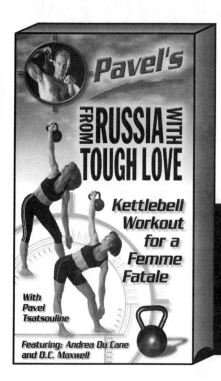

From Russia with Tough Love
Pavel's Kettlebell Workout
for a Femme Fatale
With Pavel Tsatsouline
Running Time: 1hr 12 minutes
Video #V110 $29.95
DVD #DV002 $29.95

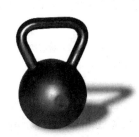

The Sure-Fire Secret to Looking Younger, Leaner and Stronger AND Having More Energy to Get a Whole Lot More Done in the Day

What you'll discover when "Tough" explodes on your monitor:

- The *Snatch*—to eliminate cellulite, firm your butt, and give you the cardio-workout of a lifetime
- The *Swing*— to fry your fat and slenderize hips 'n thighs
- The *Power Breathing Crunch*—to shrink your waist
- The *Deck Squat*— for strength and super-flexiblity
- An incredible exercise to tone your arms and shoulders
- The *Clean-and-Press*—for a magnificent upper body
- The *Overhead Squat*—for explosive leg strength
- The queen of situps—for a flat, flat stomach
- Combination exercises that wallop you with an unbelievable muscular and cardio workout

Spanking graphics, a kick-ass opening, smooth-as-silk camera work, Pavel at his absolute dynamic best, two awesome femme fatales, and a slew of fantastic KB exercises, many of which were not included on the original Russian Kettlebell Challenge video.

At one hour and twenty minutes of rock-solid, cutting-edge information, this video is value-beyond-belief. I challenge any woman worth her salt not to be able to completely transform herself physically with this one tape.

"In six weeks of kettlebell work, I lost an inch off my waist and dropped my heart rate 6 beats per minute, while staying the same weight. I was already working out when I started using kettlebells, so I'm not a novice. There are few ways to lose fat, gain muscle, and improve your cardio fitness all at the same time; I've never seen a better one than this."
—*Steven Justus, Westminster, CO*

"Kettlebells are without a doubt the most effective strength/endurance conditioning tool out there. I wish I had known about them 15 years ago!"
—*Santiago, Orlando, FL*

"I have practiced Kettlebell training for a year and a half. I now have an anatomy chart back and have gotten MUCH stronger."
—*Samantha Mendelson, Coral Gables, FL*

"I know now that I will never walk into a gym again - who would? It is absolutely amazing how much individual accomplishment can be attained using a kettlebell. Simply fantastic. I would recommend it to anyone at any fitness level, in any sport.
—*William Hevener, North Cape May, NJ*

"It is the most effective training tool I have ever used. I have increased both my speed and endurance, with extra power to boot. It wasn't even a priority, but I lost some bodyfat, which was nice. However, increased athletic performance was my main goal, and this is where the program really shines."
—*Tyler Hass, Walla Walla, WA*

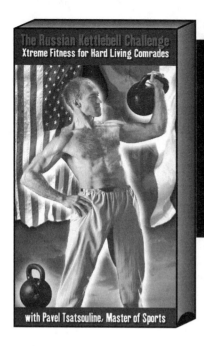

The Russian Kettlebell Challenge

Xtreme Fitness for Hard Living Comrades

with Pavel Tsatsouline, Master of Sports

Video Item # V103 • $39.95 or DVD Item # DV001 • $39.95
Running Time: 32 minutes

An ancient Russian exercise device, the kettlebell has long been a favorite in that country for those seeking a special edge in strength and endurance.

It was the key in forging the mighty power of dinosaurs like Ivan "the Champion of Champions", Poddubny. Poddubny, one of the strongest men of his time, trained with kettlebells in preparation for his undefeated wrestling career and six world champion belts.

Many famous Soviet weightlifters, such as Vorobyev, Vlasov, Alexeyev, and Stogov, started their Olympic careers with old-fashioned kettlebells.

Kettlebells come in "poods". A pood is an old Russian measure of weight, which equals 16kg, or 36 pounds. There are one, one and a half, and two pood K-bells, 16, 24, and 32kg respectively.

To earn his national ranking, Pavel Tsatsouline had to power snatch a 32kg kettlebell forty times with one arm, and forty with the other back to back and power clean and jerk two such bells forty-five times.

Soviet science discovered that repetition kettlebell lifting is one of the best tools for all around physical development. (Voropayev, 1983) observed two groups of college students over a period of a few years. A standard battery of the armed forces PT tests was used: pullups, a standing broad jump, a 100m sprint, and a 1k run. The control groupfollowed the typical university physical training program which was military oriented and emphasized the above exercises. The experimental group just lifted kettlebells. In spite of the lack of practice on the tested drills, the KB group showed better scores in every one of them.

The Red Army, too pragmatic to waste their troopers, time on pushups and situps, quickly caught on. Every Russian military unit's gym was equipped with K-bells. Spetznaz, Soviet Special Operations, personnel owe much of their wiry strength, explosive agility, and never quitting stamina to kettlebells. High rep C&Js and snatches with K-bells kick the fighting man,s system into warp drive.

In addition to their many mentioned benefits, the official kettlebell lifts also develop the ability to absorb ballistic shocks. If you want to develop your ability to take impact try the official K-bell lifts. The repetitive ballistic shock builds extremely strong tendons and ligaments.

The ballistic blasts of kettlebell lifting become an excellent conditioning tool for athletes from rough sports like kick boxing, wrestling, and football. And the extreme metabolic cost of high rep KB workouts will put your unwanted fat on a fire sale.

If you are looking for a supreme edge in your chosen sport—seek no more!

Both the Soviet Special Forces and numerous world-champion Soviet Olympic athletes used the ancient Russian Kettlebell as their secret weapon for xtreme fitness. Thanks to the kettlebells's astonishing ability to turbocharge physical performance, these Soviet supermen creamed their opponents time-and-time-again, with inhuman displays of raw power and explosive strength.

Now, former Spetznaz trainer, international fitness author and nationally ranked kettlebell lifter, Pavel Tsatsouline, delivers this secret Soviet weapon into your own hands.

You NEVER have to be second best again! Here is the first-ever complete kettlebell training program—for Western shock-attack athletes who refuse to be denied—and who'd rather be dead than number two.

- **Get really, really nasty—with a commando's wiry strength, the explosive agility of a tiger and the stamina of a world-class ironman.**

- **Own the single best conditioning tool for killer sports like kickboxing, wrestling, and football.**

- **Watch in amazement as high-rep kettlebells let you hack the fat off your meat—without the dishonor of aerobics and dieting**

- **Kick your fighting system into warp speed—with high-rep snatches and clean-and-jerks**

- **Develop steel tendons and ligaments—and a whiplash power to match**

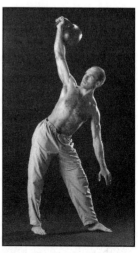

- **Effortlessly absorb ballistic shocks—and laugh as you shrug off the hardest hits your opponent can muster**

- **Go ape on your enemies—with gorilla shoulders and tree-swinging traps**

More Russian Kettlebell Challenges

25 Evil Drills for Radical Strength and Old School Toughness

With Pavel Tsatsouline

Running Time: 40 minutes

Video #V111 $59.95
DVD   #DV003 $59.95

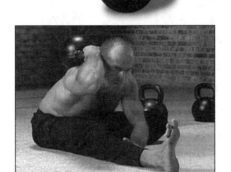

"Pavel has done another excellent job in presenting challenging drills that will take your kettlebell practice and fitness to new heights. Pavel's trademark humor is ever present, and his instruction is no-nonsense and, as always, well done. Multiple camera angles are used, and are very helpful in grasping the fine points of the drills. Pavel's instruction is pure gold — detailed and meticulous. There is a tremendous amount of valuable information packed into this 40-minute tape. Watch and listen closely, follow Pavel's advice, and you'll find something remarkable in the fitness industry — someone actually delivering on what might appear to be the usual marketing hyperbole."—John Quigley, Hazleton, PA

"The video takes you through some new moves with great detail and also revisits some older ones with more attention to the finer points. This tape will give you many more weapons in your arsenal of KB exercises. KB's offer variety of exercises and great flexibility in program design and this video will give you more to work with. Highly recommended!"—Dave Randolph, RKC, Louisville, KY

"Pavel Tsatsouline delivers some outstanding instruction that has to be seen to be appreciated. Do your self a favor and get this video. The quality is what you would expect of a Tsatsouline video. The drills are demonstrated with adept skill and perfect execution. He is an example that this stuff works. 25 drills in this video. Some of them expand on the ones previously demonstrated in the "Russian Kettlebell Challenge",

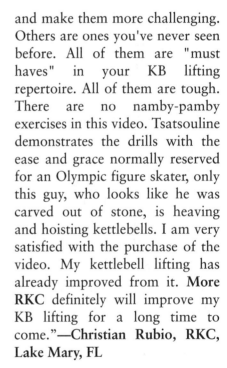

and make them more challenging. Others are ones you've never seen before. All of them are "must haves" in your KB lifting repertoire. All of them are tough. There are no namby-pamby exercises in this video. Tsatsouline demonstrates the drills with the ease and grace normally reserved for an Olympic figure skater, only this guy, who looks like he was carved out of stone, is heaving and hoisting kettlebells. I am very satisfied with the purchase of the video. My kettlebell lifting has already improved from it. **More RKC definitely will improve my KB lifting for a long time to come.**"—**Christian Rubio, RKC, Lake Mary, FL**

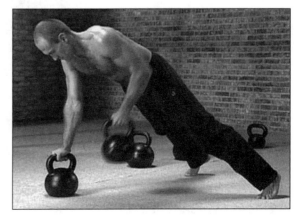

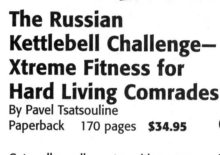
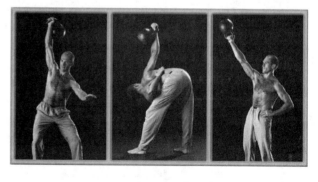

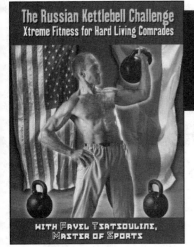

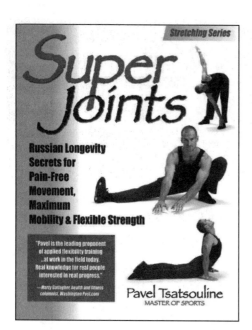

Super Joints #B16

Russian Longevity Secrets for Pain-Free Movement, Maximum Mobility & Flexible Strength
Book By Pavel Tsatsouline
Paperback 130 pages 8.5" x 11"
Over 100 photos and illustrations

#B16 $34.95

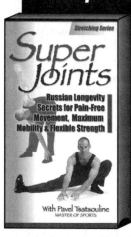

Super Joints
Video
With Pavel Tsatsouline
Running Time 33 minutes

#V108 $24.95

#V108

"The Do-It-Now, Fast-Start, Get-Up-and-Go, Jump-into-Action Bible for HIGH PERFORMANCE and LONGER LIFE"

You have a choice in life. You can sputter and stumble and creak your way along in a process of painful, slow decline—or you can take charge of your health and become a human dynamo.

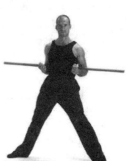

And there is no better way to insure a long, pain-free life than performing the right daily combination of joint mobility and strength-flexibility exercises.

In *Super Joints*, Russian fitness expert Pavel Tsatsouline shows you exactly how to quickly achieve and maintain peak joint health—and then use it to improve every aspect of your physical performance.

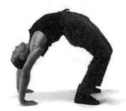

Only the foolish would deliberately ignore the life-saving and life-enhancing advice Pavel offers in *Super Joints*. Why would anyone willingly subject themselves to a life of increasing pain, degeneration and decrepitude? But for an athlete, a dancer, a martial artist or any serious performer, *Super Joints* could spell the difference between greatness and mediocrity.

Discover:

- The twenty-eight most valuable drills for youthful joints and a stronger stretch
- How to save your joints and prevent or reduce arthritis
- The one-stop care-shop for your inner Tin Man—how to give your nervous system a tune up, your joints a lube-job and your energy a recharge
- What it takes to go from cruise control to full throttle: The One Thousand Moves Morning Recharge Amosov's "bigger bang" calisthenics complex for achieving heaven-on earth in 25 minutes
- How to make your body feel better than you can remember—active flexibility fosporting prowess and fewer injuries
- The amazing Pink Panther technique that may add a couple of feet to your stretch the first time you do it

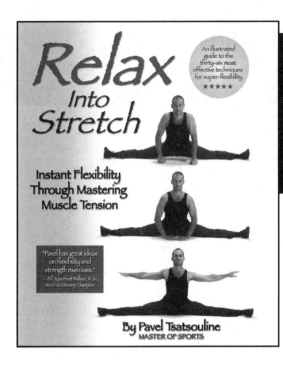

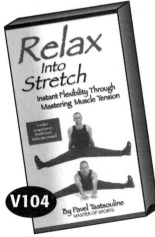
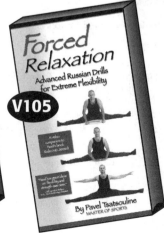

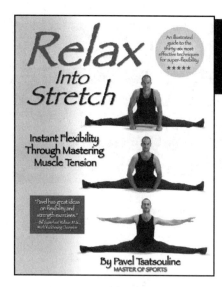

Relax into Stretch

Instant Flexibility Through Mastering Muscle Tension

By Pavel Tsatsouline

$34.95

Stretching is NOT the best way to become flexible

Why Americans lose flexibility as they grow older • the dangers of physically stretching muscles and ligaments • *the role of antagonist passive insufficiency* • the nature and function of the *stretch reflex* • how to master muscular tension •
how to inhibit the stretch reflex • intensive and extensive learning methods.

Waiting out the Tension— relaxed stretching as it should be

Just relax—when and when not to use the technique of *Waiting out the Tension* • Victor Popenko's key to mobility • the importance of visualization • why fear and anxiety reduce your flexibility • maximizing perceived safety in the stretch.

Proprioceptive Neuromuscular Facilitation

How Kabat's PNF fools your stretch reflex • the function of the *Renshaw cell* • why it works to pre-tense a stretched muscle.

Isometric stretching rules!

Why contract-relax stretching is 267% more effective than conventional relaxed stretching • what the 'frozen shoulder' has to teach us • the lifestyle problem of *'tight weakness'*, • why isometrics is more practical than weights.

Extreme flexibility through *Contrast Breathing*

How to breathe your way to greater flexibility • effective visualizations for the tension/release sequence • avoiding the dangers of hyperventilation.

Forced Relaxation— the Russian spirit of stretching

How to turn the contract-relax approach into a thermonuclear stretching weapon • determining correct duration • tips for the correct release of tension.

The final frontier: why *Clasp Knife* stretches will work when everything else fails

How to cancel out the *stretch reflex* • taking advantage of the *inverse stretch reflex* • the last line of defense against injuries • shutdown threshold isometrics • mastering the Golgi tendon reflex.

Why you should not stretch your ligaments— and how you can tell if you are

Yoga postures and stretches to avoid at all costs • the function and limitations of your ligaments.

Stretching when injured

Rest, Ice, Compression and Elevation • what happens when a muscle gets injured • contracting and releasing the injury • why stretching won't help a bad back and what to do instead.

The demographics of stretching

Why your age and sex should determine your stretches • the best—and worst—stretches for young girls, boys and adolescents • a warning for pregnant women • what's best for older folks.

The details, the schedule

Isometric stretches—when to do them and how often • how to know if you are doing too much • Bill 'Superfoot' Wallace's hardcore stretching schedule • correct order and choice of stretch • why isometric stretching should be the last exercise you do in your day.

The *Relax into Stretch* drills—

How much flexibility do you really need?

Why excessive flexibility can be detrimental to athletic performance • why old school strongmen instinctively avoided stretching • what stretches powerlifters and weightlifters do and don't need • warning examples from sprinting, boxing and kickboxing.

When flexibility is hard to come by, build strength

Plateau-busting strategies for the chronically inflexible • *high total time under tension.*

Two more plateau busting strategies from the iron world

Popenko's flexibility data • the reminiscence effect • the dynamic stereotype • How to exceed your old limits with the stepwise progression.

Advanced Russian Drills for Extreme Flexibility—

Discover incredibly simple ways to eliminate threats to your well being and enjoy amazing, life-long health

The Fit For Life Solution

How to Identify and Successfully Eradicate The Causes of Pain, Fatigue and Disease— NOW!

8 1/2" x 11" Paperback 336 pages • Over 50 photos and illustrations

Item # B19 $24.00

Deluxe Edition of *Fit for Life: A New Beginning*

The ALL-NATURAL, DRUG-FREE WAY to A WONDERFUL LIFE of RADIANT HEALTH

"An empowering resource...*The Fit For Life Solution* really delivers."
—Anthony Robbins

"*The Fit For Life Solution* is a book with answers, a book of real hope...a treasure trove of exciting health information to prevent disease."
—Kenneth M. Kroll, M.D., International College of Surgeons

"Bravo! Harvey Diamond has done it again. He clearly reveals how we can take charge of our own health and prevent disease."
—Dr. Wayne Dyer, Author of Manifest Your Destiny: *The Nine Spiritual Principles for Everything You Want* and *Your Erroneous Zones*

"Harvey Diamond gives everyone a powerful tool for the restoration of health. He speaks from a point of view so many of us now want: with an awareness of nature, consciousness and their role in healing. I deeply welcome this book into my own life."
—Marianne Williamson, Author of *A Return to Love; Woman's Worth; Illuminata*

Is it possible to enjoy a life without pain? Without disease? Without obesity? With energy to spare? And all-around vibrant health? The answer is a resounding YES! With Harvey Diamond's revolutionary new book, *THE FIT FOR LIFE SOLUTION*, a truly healthy life is yours for the taking.

Discover the simple but astoundingly effective three-step CARE program to:

- **Easily lose all the weight you want...forever!**
- **Understand and prevent the seven stages of disease**
- **Quickly cleanse your lymph system of the toxins that make you sick**
- **Avoid all cancers with confidence**
- **Always know what's best to minimize and maximize in your diet**
- **Dramatically boost your energy**
- **Magically eliminate digestive problems, headaches, and other chronic pain**

- **Avoid Cancer**
- **Live Pain-Free**
- **Evade Life-Threatening Conditions**
- **Lose Weight and Keep it Off Forever**
- **Bounce with New-Found Energy**
- **Look and Feel Terrific—All the Time**

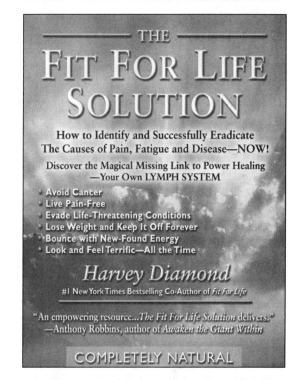

About Harvey Diamond

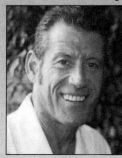

Harvey Diamond is the co-author of the #1 *New York Times* bestseller, *Fit for Life*, which has sold over 11 million copies worldwide and has been translated into 32 languages.

Internationally known as an author, teacher, and health consultant, he has appeared on hundreds of radio and TV programs including *Larry King Live!*, *Oprah!*, *Nightline*, and *Good Morning America*.

He lives in Sarasota, Florida.

Manage Stress, Reduce Pain, Restore Energy, and Heal Yourself with the HIGHLY EFFECTIVE and PLEASURABLE METHODS of Chinese QIGONG

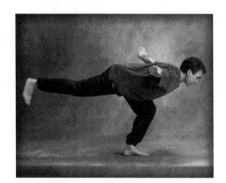

"John Du Cane has taken an ancient Chinese system, developed almost 2,000 years ago, and put together a practical and workable Qigong program for today's modern lifestyles. The Five Animals Frolics Qigong system is a series of exercises developed by ancient physicians that combines principles of Chinese medicine with shamanic healing systems. Its goal is to combine a wide range of movement, special breathing patterns, and visualization to awaken the internal power of self-healing. John Du Cane gives a strong demonstration of The Five Animals Frolics and clear instruction on each of these exercises that is beneficial to those beginning Qigong, as well as to seasoned practitioners."

—Rob Bracco, Editorial review for Amazon.com

"John Du Cane has created a good tape for learning some basic qigong practices. The instruction is clear and easily understood. The Bliss qigong movements are clearly explained in this tape, and are appropriate for beginners or experienced practitioners. Instructions are given in a logical fashion and at a pace that anyone can follow. His teaching style is gentle and the movements are not difficult to learn. His delivery is even and his manner inspires confidence. Along with teaching the movements, he includes information about qi and how it feels and functions in context of the exercises. There is not a lot of flash and glitter in the presentation, just straightforward instruction as if you were in the room with your teacher. This tape is easily among the best I have seen in the genre, and I would not hesitate to buy more of John Du Cane's works. I find the quality of his instruction to be in the same league as that of Ken Cohen and Chunyi Lin."

—Jon Norris, La Grande, OR

"One of the keys to success in life (as well as combat) is the ability to stay relaxed and focused. Many people struggle with this issue. I have seen people who are great practice athletes, but when competition time arrives, they become their worst nightmare. They get nervous and don't know how to channel this energy. The same is true in almost any endeavor.

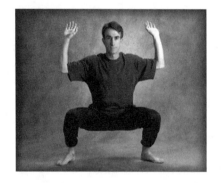

Knowing how to channel nervous energy is a skill, and so is keeping your body relaxed. Even while you're reading this message, I'm sure most of you are using muscles that don't need to be doing anything. I'm also sure that most of you aren't breathing as deeply as you could be or should be. One thing that I have greatly benefited from over the years is the study of qigong or deep breathing exercises. I have done these exercises while holding still postures and I have done them while moving. It doesn't matter which way you do them, all that matters is that you are moving the energy in your body while staying relaxed and focused.

Recently I watched a NEW set of videotapes, produced by John Du Cane, on what is called "Five Animal Frolics Qigong." I tried to watch the tapes first to get an idea of what was on them, but it didn't take long for me to stop watching and start participating. Watching how gracefully John moved from one position to the next, and how relaxed he was, really got me thinking about how I needed to improve upon this skill as well. I especially liked the set of movements based upon the bear and the monkey. Really awesome. These movements generate POWER, that's for sure.

I highly recommend these tapes. Find out how to relax, reduce stress, increase power and energy, eliminate aches and pains, increase circulation and so on."

—Matt Furey, author of Combat Conditioning

Five Animal Frolics Workbook

Detailed descriptions of postural alignment, movement, breathing and use of attention combine with a wealth of photographs to provide an easy-learning tool for the world's most famous qigong system.

Five Animal Frolics   #B12
By John Du Cane
8 1/2" x 11" Spiralbound workbook, 110 pages.
100 photographs, Item #B12   **$29.95**

The Five Animal Frolics

A Form Workbook
By John Du Cane

A Complete Qigong Program for High Energy, Vitality and Well Being

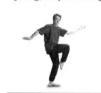

About John Du Cane

John began his Qigong and Tai Chi practice in 1975. John has developed and presented national certification training programs for medical qigong. He has presented on qigong at the Arnold Schwarzenegger Martial Arts Fitness Seminar and taught at Northwestern Health Sciences University, the Institute for Renewing Community Leadership, Minnesota Center for Shiatsu Studies, The Open U and Newbridge Wellness Center.

"I felt completely CENTERED, FOCUSED, RELAXED and at PEACE, all accompanied by a VIBRANT SENSE OF ENERGY and WELL BEING."

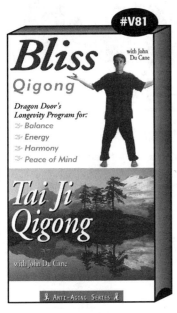

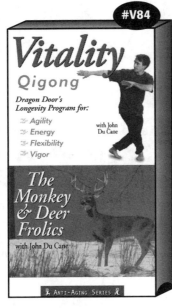

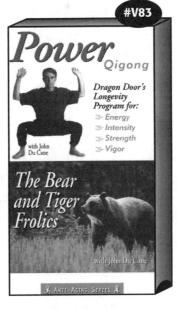

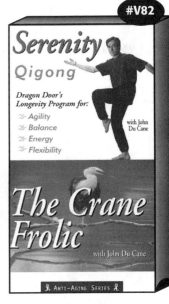

BLISS QIGONG
An instructional guide to Tai Ji Qigong

 # V81. 54 minutes. $29.95

Reveals the Yang Family's personal qigong program, with additional tips on energy accumulation and balancing. The simple movements gently harmonize the qi, promote blood circulation, cultivate vitality, regulate the breath and reduce stress.

Discover:
- How to use attention to effectively feel and direct qi
- How to activate all your major energy centers
- How to turn on healing power in your hands
- How to clear all the major meridians in your body
- How to develop your sensing ability
- How to get real results with you standing qigong practice
- How to incorporate special internal sounds to deepen your meditation

VITALITY QIGONG
An instructional guide to The Monkey and Deer Frolics

 # V84. 43 minutes. $29.95

The Monkey develops suppleness, agility, and quick wit, training you to remain alert and calm, even as you are outwardly spirited and mobile. The Deer gives a long stretch to the legs and spine, creating open, expansive movement with very flexible sinews and bones. The Deer embodies grace and relaxation, while regulating the endocrine system.

Discover:
- How to flood your system with warming qi
- How to quickly improve your muscle tone
- How to develop strong, mobile joints

POWER QIGONG
An instructional guide to The Bear and Tiger Frolics

 # V83. 48 minutes. $29.95

The Bear is a great winter exercise. Slow, ponderous, but very strong, it warms the body, strengthens the spleen, and builds vitality. The Bear's twisting waist movements massage and invigorate the kidneys. The Bear is an excellent preventive against osteoporosis, as it is known to fortify the bones. The dynamic Tiger builds great power, strengthening your waist, sinews, and kidneys and developing you internally.

Discover:
- How to develop power and strength
- How to generate coiling energy
- How to develop a strong root

SERENITY QIGONG
An instructional guide to The Crane Frolic

 # V82. 41 minutes. $29.95

Practice an invigorating mix of dynamic and tranquil postures for self-healing and athletic grace. The Crane develops balance, lightness, and agility, releases the spine, and relaxes your whole body.

Discover:
- How to absorb qi from the universe for self-healing
- How to extend your qi beyond your own body
- How to develop balanced leg strength
- How to heal your lungs

1. Improve your metabolism, digestion, and elimination—for weight control, more youthful appearance, and **higher, longer-lasting energy.**

2. Stimulate the lymph system—for a **stronger immune system.** Be less susceptible to the flu or colds and recover faster if you do get sick.

3. Improve your circulation—alleviating conditions such as arthritis and chronic fatigue.

4. Build **stronger, more durable bones.**

5. Give your internal organs an "inner massage"—retarding the aging process by restoring your organs to peak efficiency.

6. Increase oxygen in the tissues—reducing tensions, blocks and stagnant energy.

7. Lubricate the joints—for **pain free movement and greater flexibility.**

8. Soothe the nervous system—for feelings of contentment and serenity.

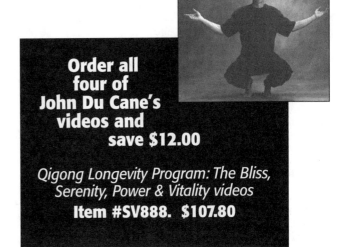

Order all four of John Du Cane's videos and save $12.00

Qigong Longevity Program: The Bliss, Serenity, Power & Vitality videos

Item #SV888. $107.80

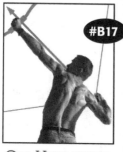

The Warrior Diet
How to Take Advantage of
Undereating and Overeating
Nature's Ultimate Secret for Burning Fat,
Igniting Energy and Boosting Brain Power
By Ori Hofmekler
With Diana Holtzberg

Hardcover 5 3/8" x 8 3/8", 420 pages,
Over 150 photographs and illustrations
Item #B17   **$26.95**

Eat like an emperor—and have a gladiator's body

Are you still confused about what, how and when to eat? Despite the diet books you have read and the programs you have tried, do you still find yourself lacking in energy, carrying excess body fat, and feeling physically run-down? Sexually, do you feel a shadow of your former self?

The problem, according to **Ori Hofmekler,** is that we have lost touch with the natural wisdom of our instinctual drives. We have become the slaves of our own creature comforts—scavenger/victims rather than predator/victors. When to comes to informed-choice, we lack any real sense of personal freedom. The result: ill-advised eating and lifestyle habits that leave us vulnerable to all manner of disease—not to mention obesity and sub-par performance.

The Warrior Diet presents a brilliant and far-reaching solution to our nutritional woes, based on a return to the primal power of our natural instincts.

The first step is to break the chains of our current eating habits. Drawing on a combination of ancient history and modern science, *The Warrior Diet* proves that humans are at their energetic, physical, mental and passionate best when they "undereat" during the day and "overeat" at night. Once you master this essential eating cycle, a new life of explosive vigor and vitality will be yours for the taking.

Unlike so many dietary gurus, Ori Hofmekler has personally followed his diet for over twenty-five years and is a perfect model of *the Warrior Diet's* success—the man is a human dynamo.

Not just a diet, but a whole way of life, *the Warrior Diet* encourages us to seize back the pleasures of being alive—from the most refined to the wild and raw. *The Warrior Diet* is practical, tested, and based in commonsense. Expect results!

The Warrior Diet covers all the bases. As an added bonus, discover delicious Warrior Recipes, a special Warrior Workout, and a line of Warrior Supplements—designed to give you every advantage in the transformation of your life from average to exceptional.

About Ori Hofmekler

Ori Hofmekler is a modern Renaissance man whose life has been driven by two passions: art and sports. Hofmekler's formative experience as a young man with the Israeli Special Forces, prompted a lifetime's interest in diets and fitness regimes that would optimize his physical and mental performance.

After the army, Ori attended the Bezalel Academy of Art and the Hebrew University, where he studied art and philosophy and received a degree in Human Sciences.

A world-renowned painter, best known for his controversial political satire, Ori's work has been featured in magazines worldwide, including *Time, Newsweek, Rolling Stone, People, The New Republic* as well as *Penthouse* where he was a monthly columnist for 17 years and Health Editor from 1998–2000. Ori has published two books of political art, *Hofmekler's People,* and *Hofmekler's Gallery.*

As founder, Editor-In-Chief, and Publisher of *Mind & Muscle Power,* a national men's health and fitness magazine, Ori introduced his Warrior Diet to the public in a monthly column—to immediate acclaim from readers and professionals in the health industry alike.

NUTRITION AND FITNESS EXPERTS IN STAMPEDE TO ENDORSE BENEFITS OF THE WARRIOR DIET

"In my quest for a lean, muscular body, I have seen practically every diet and suffered through most of them. It is also my business to help others with their fat loss programs. I am supremely skeptical of any eating plan or "diet" book that can't tell me how and why it works in simple language. Ori Hofmekler's *The Warrior Diet* does just this, with a logical, readable approach that provides grounding for his claims and never asks the reader to take a leap of faith. *The Warrior Diet* can be a very valuable weapon in the personal arsenal of any woman."

—DC Maxwell, 2-time Women's Brazilian Jiu-Jitsu World Champion, Co-Owner, Maxercise Sports/Fitness Training Center and Relson Gracie Jiu-Jitsu Academy East

"The credo that has served me well in my life and that which I tell my patients is that I only take advice from those who practice what they preach. To me, there is nothing more pathetic and laughable than to see the terrible physical condition of many of the self-proclaimed diet and fitness experts of today. Those hypocrites who do not live by their own words are not worth your time, or mine.

At the other extreme, Ori Hofmekler is the living, breathing example of a warrior. There is real strength in the sinews of his muscle. There is wisdom and power in his words. His passion for living honestly is intense and reflective of the toil of a tough army life. Yet in a fascinating and true Spartan way, his physical nature is tempered by an equal reveling in the love of art, knowledge of the classic poets, and in the drinking of fine wine with good conversation.

Welcome *The Warrior Diet* into your life and you usher in the honest and real values of a man who has truly walked the walk. He has treaded the dirt of the path that lay before you, and is thus a formidable guide to a new beginning. He is your shepherd of integrity that will lead you out of the bondage of misinformation. His approach is what I call "revolutionarily de-evolutionary". In other words, your freedom from excess body fat, flat energy levels, and poor physical performance begins with unlearning the modern ways, which have failed you, and forging a new understanding steeped in the secret traditions of the ancient Roman warrior."

—Carlon M. Colker, M.D., F.A.C.N., author of *The Greenwich Diet*, CEO and Medical Director, Peak Wellness, Inc.

"*The Warrior Diet* certainly defies so-called modern nutritional and training dogmas. Having met Ori on several occasions, I can certainly attest that he is the living proof that his system works. He maintains a ripped muscular body year round despite juggling extreme workloads and family life. His take on supplementation is refreshing as he promotes an integrated and timed approach. *The Warrior Diet* is a must read for the nutrition and training enthusiast who wishes to expand his horizons."

—Charles Poliquin, author of *The Poliquin Principles* and *Modern Trends in Strength Training*, Three-Time Olympic Strength Coach

"Despite its name, *The Warrior Diet* isn't about leading a Spartan lifestyle, although it is about improving quality of life. With a uniquely compelling approach, the book guides you towards the body you want by re-awakening primal instinct and biofeedback—the things that have allowed us to evolve this far.

Ironically, in a comfortable world of overindulgence, your survival may still be determined by natural selection. If this is the case, *The Warrior Diet* will be the only tool you'll need."

—Brian Batcheldor, Science writer/researcher, National Coach, British Powerlifting Team

"In a era of decadence, where wants and desires are virtually limitless, Ori's vision recalls an age of warriors, where success meant survival and survival was the only option. A diet of the utmost challenge from which users will reap tremendous benefits."

—John Davies, Olympic and professional sports strength/speed coach

"Ori Hofmekler has his finger on a deep, ancient and very visceral pulse—one that too many of us have all but forgotten. Part warrior-athlete, part philosopher-romantic, Ori not only reminds us what this innate, instinctive rhythm is all about, he also shows us how to detect and rekindle it in our own bodies. His program challenges and guides each of us to fully reclaim for ourselves the strength, sinew, energy and spirit that humans have always been meant to possess."

—Pilar Gerasimo, Editor in Chief, *Experience Life Magazine*

"Ori and I became friends and colleagues in 1997 when he so graciously took me under his wing as a writer for *Penthouse* Magazine and *Mind and Muscle Power*.

When I received *The Warrior Diet* in the mail I nearly burst with pride. Not only because my dear friend had finally reached his particular goal of helping others be the best they can be physically, but because I had a small role in the creation of the book. Ori enlisted my help in researching topics such as the benefits of fasting, the perfect protein, and glycogen loading. I believe in Ori's concepts because I trust him wholeheartedly and because I helped uncover the scientific data that proves them. I also live by *The Warrior Diet*, although not to the extreme that Ori does. My body continues to get tighter and more toned in all of the right places...and people marvel at my eating practices.

1·800·899·5111
24 HOURS A DAY
FAX YOUR ORDER (866) 280-7619

Read *The Warrior Diet* with an open mind. Digest the information at your own pace. Assimilate the knowledge to make it fit into your current lifestyle. You will be amazed at how much more productive and energetic you will be. Be a warrior in your own right. Your body will thank you for it."

—Laura Moore, Science writer, *Penthouse* Magazine, *IronMan* Magazine, Body of the Month for IronMan, Sept 2001, Radio Talk Show Host *The Health Nuts*, author of *Sex Heals*

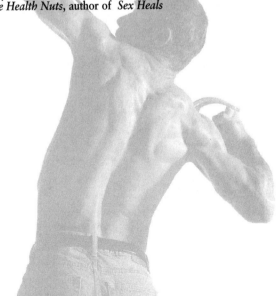

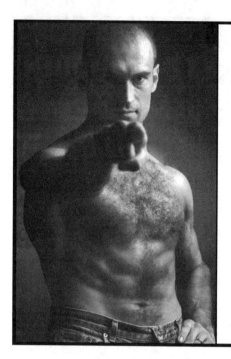
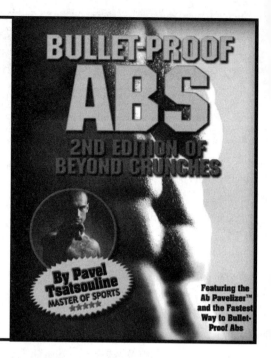

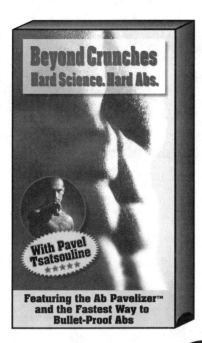

Beyond Crunches
Hard Science. Hard Abs.

With Pavel Tsatsouline
★★★★★

Featuring the Ab Pavelizer™
and the Fastest Way to
Bullet-Proof Abs

BEYOND #V90
CRUNCHES
By Pavel Tsatsouline

Video, Running time: 37 min

$29.95   #V90

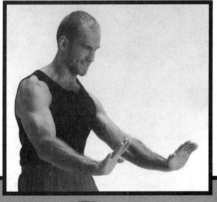
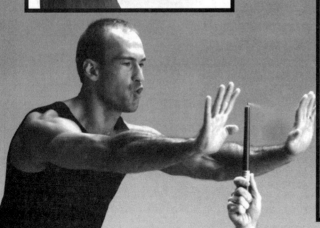
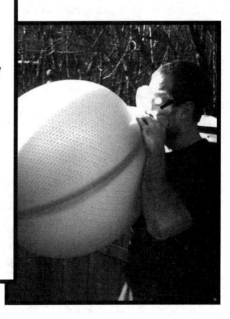

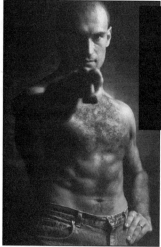

"New Ab Machine Exposes Frauds, Fakes and Cheaters—But Rewards Faithful with the Most Spectacular Abs This Side of Heaven"

The Ab Pavelizer™ II
Item # P12

$130.00
10-25 lb Olympic plate required for correct use.
(You will need to supply your own plate)

#P12

You know, it's a crying shame to cheat on your abs. Your abs are your very core, your center. Your abs define you, man or woman. So why betray them with neglect and less-than-honest carryings-on? That's bad! And everybody always knows! Rationalize all you want, hide all you want, but weak, flabby abs scream your lack of self-respect to all comers. Why live at all, if you can't hold your head up high and own a flat stomach?

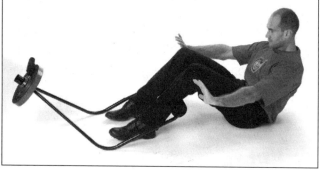

Fortunately, you can now come clean, get honest and give your abs the most challenging, yet rewarding workout of their lives. And believe me, they will love you for ever!

Maybe you've been misled. Maybe you think you have to flog out hundreds of situps to get spectacular abs? Ho! Sorry, **but with abs, repetition is the mother of insanity.** Forget about it! You're just wasting your time! You're just fooling around! No wonder you're still not satisfied!

No, if you really, really want abs-to-die-for then: INTENSITY IS EVERYTHING!

FREE BONUS:

Comes with a four page detailed instruction guide on how to use and get the most out of your Ab Pavelizer™ II. Includes two incredible methods for massively intensifying your ab workout with *Power* and *Paradox Breathing*.

And here lies the secret of **The Ab Pavelizer™ II**. It's all in the extreme, unavoidable intensity it thrusts on you. No room for skulkers or shirkers. No room at all! Either get with the program or slink back under the stone from under which you crept.

You see, The Ab Pavelizer™ II's new sleek-'n-light design guarantees a perfect sit-up by forcing you to do it right. Now, escape or half-measures are impossible. Sit down at the Ab Pavelizer™ II and a divine slab of abs will be served up whether you like it or not. You'll startle yourself in your own mirror!

The secret to the Ab Pavelizer™ II is in the extra-active resistance it provides you. The cunning device literally pushes up against your calves (you'd almost swear it was a cruel, human partner) and forces you to recruit your glutes and hamstrings.

Two wonderful and amazing things happen.

First, it is virtually impossible to do the Janda situp wrong unless you start with a jerk. Second, the exercise becomes MUCH harder than on the Ab Pavelizer™ Classic. And "Much Harder" is Russian for "Quicker Results."

It is astonishingly hard to sit up all the way when the new Ab Pavelizer™ II is loaded with enough weight, 10-35 pounds for most comrades. If you can do three sets of five reps you will already have awesome abs.

A Great Added Benefit: Are you living in an already over-cluttered space? Want to conveniently hide the secret of your abs-success from envious neighbors? The new Ab Pavelizer™ II easily and quickly folds away in a closet or under your bed. Once prying eyes have left, you can put it up again in seconds for another handshake with heaven—or hell, depending on your perspective.

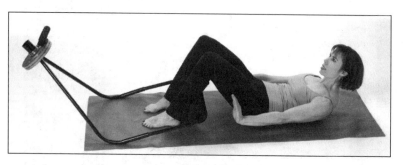

1•800•899•5111 24 HOURS A DAY, OR FAX: (866) 280-7619

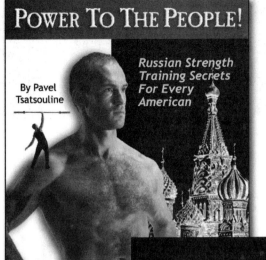

POWER TO THE PEOPLE!

RUSSIAN STRENGTH TRAINING SECRETS FOR EVERY AMERICAN

By Pavel Tsatsouline

8½" x 11" 124 pages, over 100 photographs and illustrations—$34.95 #B10

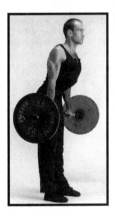

How would you like to own a world class body—<u>whatever your present condition</u>— by doing only two exercises, for twenty minutes a day?" A body so lean, ripped and powerful looking, you won't believe your own reflection when you catch yourself in the mirror.

And what if you could do it without a single supplement, without having to waste your time at a gym and with only a 150 bucks of simple equipment?

And how about not only being stronger than you've ever been in your life, but having higher energy and better performance in whatever you do?

How would you like to have an instant download of the world's <u>absolutely most effective strength secrets?</u> To possess exactly the same knowledge that created world-champion athletes—and the strongest bodies of their generation?"

Pavel Tsatsouline's *Power to the People!– Russian Strength Training Secrets for Every American* delivers all of this and more.

As Senior Science Editor for Joe Weider's *Flex* magazine, Jim Wright is recognized as one of the world's premier authorities on strength training. Here's more of what he had to say:

And how about this from World Masters Powerlifting champion and Parrillo Performance Press editor, Marty Gallagher:

Here's just some of what you'll discover, when you possess your own copy of Pavel Tsatsouline's *Power to the People!*:

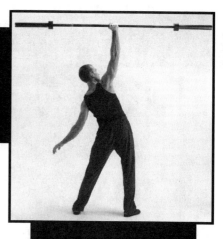

- How to get super strong without training to muscle failure or exhaustion
- How to hack into your 'muscle software' and magnify your power and muscle definition
- How to get super strong <u>without putting on an ounce of weight</u>
- Or how to build massive muscles with a classified Soviet Special Forces workout
- Why high rep training to the 'burn' is like a form of rigor mortis—and what it really takes to develop spectacular muscle tone
- How to mold your whole body into an off-planet rock with only two exercises
- How to increase your bench press by ten pounds overnight
- How to get a tremendous workout on the road without any equipment
- How to design a world class body in your basement—with $150 worth of basic weights and in twenty minutes a day
- How futuristic techniques can squeeze more horsepower out of your body-engine
- How to maximize muscular tension for traffic-stopping muscular definition
- How to minimize fatigue and get the most out of your strength training
- How to ensure high energy after your workout
- How to get stronger and harder without getting bigger
- Why it's safer to use free weights than machines
- How to achieve massive muscles <u>and</u> awesome strength—if that's what you want
- What, how and when to eat for maximum gains
- How to master the magic of effective exercise variation
- The ultimate formula for strength
- How to gain beyond your wildest dreams—with less chance of injury
- A high intensity, immediate gratification technique for massive strength gains
- The eight most effective breathing habits for lifting weights
- The secret that separates elite athletes from 'also-rans'
- How to become super strong and live to tell about it

"You are not training if you are not training with Pavel!"

—Dr. Fred Clary, National Powerlifting Champion and World Record Holder.

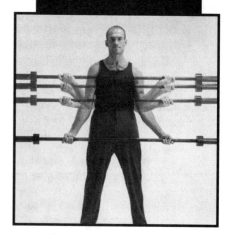

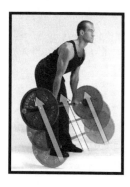

Russians have always made do with simple solutions without compromising the results. NASA aerospace types say that while America sends men to the moon in a Cadillac, Russia manages to launch them into space in a tin can. Enter the tin can approach to designing a world class body—in your basement with $150 worth of equipment. After all, US gyms are stuffed with hi-tech gear, yet it is the Russians with their metal junkyard training facilities who have dominated the Olympics for decades.

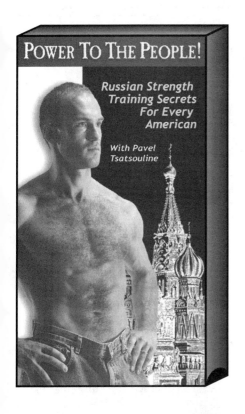
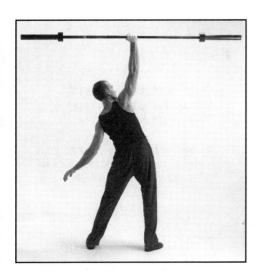

ORDERING INFORMATION

Customer Service Questions? Please call us between 9:00am–11:00pm EST Monday to Friday at 1-800-899-5111. Local and foreign customers call 513-346-4160 for orders and customer service

100% One-Year Risk-Free Guarantee. If you are not completely satisfied with any product–for any reason, no matter how long after you received it–we'll be happy to give you a prompt exchange, credit, or refund, as you wish. Simply return your purchase to us, and please let us know why you were dissatisfied–it will help us to provide better products and services in the future. *Shipping and handling fees are non-refundable.*

Telephone Orders For faster service you may place your orders by calling Toll Free 24 hours a day, 7 days a week, 365 days per year. When you call, please have your credit card ready.

1·800·899·5111
24 HOURS A DAY
FAX YOUR ORDER (866) 280-7619

Complete and mail with full payment to: Dragon Door Publications, P.O. Box 1097, West Chester, OH 45071

Please print clearly

Sold To: **A**

Name_____

Street_____

City_____

State_____ Zip_____

Day phone*_____
* Important for clarifying questions on orders

Please print clearly

SHIP TO: *(Street address for delivery)* **B**

Name_____

Street_____

City_____

State_____ Zip_____

Email_____

ITEM #	QTY.	ITEM DESCRIPTION	ITEM PRICE	A OR B	TOTAL

HANDLING AND SHIPPING CHARGES • NO COD'S

Total Amount of Order Add:

$00.00 to $24.99	add	$5.00	$100.00 to $129.99 add	$12.00
$25.00 to $39.99	add	$6.00	$130.00 to $169.99 add	$14.00
$40.00 to $59.99	add	$7.00	$170.00 to $199.99 add	$16.00
$60.00 to $99.99	add	$10.00	$200.00 to $299.99 add	$18.00
			$300.00 and up add	$20.00

Canada & Mexico add $8.00. All other countries triple U.S. charges.

Total of Goods	
Shipping Charges	
Rush Charges	
Kettlebell Shipping Charges	
OH residents add 6% sales tax	
MN residents add 6.5% sales tax	
TOTAL ENCLOSED	

METHOD OF PAYMENT ❏ CHECK ❏ M.O. ❏ MASTERCARD ❏ VISA ❏ DISCOVER   ❏ AMEX

Account No. *(Please indicate all the numbers on your credit card)*   EXPIRATION DATE

▢▢▢▢ ▢▢▢▢ ▢▢▢▢ ▢▢▢▢   ▢▢/▢▢

Day Phone (   )_____

SIGNATURE _____ DATE _____

NOTE: We ship best method available for your delivery address. Foreign orders are sent by air. Credit card or International M.O. only. For rush processing of your order, add an additional $10.00 per address. Available on money order & charge card orders only.

Errors and omissions excepted. Prices subject to change without notice.

DDP 04/03

ORDERING INFORMATION

Customer Service Questions? Please call us between 9:00am–11:00pm EST Monday to Friday at 1-800-899-5111. Local and foreign customers call 513-346-4160 for orders and customer service

100% One-Year Risk-Free Guarantee. If you are not completely satisfied with any product–for any reason, no matter how long after you received it–we'll be happy to give you a prompt exchange, credit, or refund, as you wish. Simply return your purchase to us, and please let us know why you were dissatisfied–it will help us to provide better products and services in the future. *Shipping and handling fees are non-refundable.*

Telephone Orders For faster service you may place your orders by calling Toll Free 24 hours a day, 7 days a week, 365 days per year. When you call, please have your credit card ready.

1·800·899·5111
24 HOURS A DAY
FAX YOUR ORDER (866) 280-7619

Complete and mail with full payment to: Dragon Door Publications, P.O. Box 1097, West Chester, OH 45071

Please print clearly

Sold To: **A**

Name_____

Street_____

City_____

State _____ Zip _____

Day phone*_____
Important for clarifying questions on orders

Please print clearly

SHIP TO: *(Street address for delivery)* **B**

Name_____

Street_____

City_____

State _____ Zip _____

Email_____

ITEM #	QTY.	ITEM DESCRIPTION	ITEM PRICE	A OR B	TOTAL

HANDLING AND SHIPPING CHARGES • NO COD'S
Total Amount of Order Add:

$00.00 to $24.99 add $5.00	$100.00 to $129.99 add $12.00
$25.00 to $39.99 add $6.00	$130.00 to $169.99 add $14.00
$40.00 to $59.99 add $7.00	$170.00 to $199.99 add $16.00
$60.00 to $99.99 add $10.00	$200.00 to $299.99 add $18.00
	$300.00 and up add $20.00

Canada & Mexico add $8.00. All other countries triple U.S. charges.

Total of Goods	
Shipping Charges	
Rush Charges	
Kettlebell Shipping Charges	
OH residents add 6% sales tax	
MN residents add 6.5% sales tax	
TOTAL ENCLOSED	

METHOD OF PAYMENT ❏ CHECK ❏ M.O. ❏ MASTERCARD ❏ VISA ❏ DISCOVER ❏ AMEX

Account No. *(Please indicate all the numbers on your credit card)*   EXPIRATION DATE

□□□□ □□□□ □□□□ □□□□   □□/□□

Day Phone ( ) _____

SIGNATURE _____ DATE _____

NOTE: *We ship best method available for your delivery address. Foreign orders are sent by air. Credit card or International M.O. only. For rush processing of your order, add an additional $10.00 per address. Available on money order & charge card orders only.*

Errors and omissions excepted. Prices subject to change without notice.

Warning to foreign customers:
The Customs in your country may or may not tax or otherwise charge you an additional fee for goods you receive. Dragon Door Publications is charging you only for U.S. handling and international shipping. Dragon Door Publications is in no way responsible for any additional fees levied by Customs, the carrier or any other entity.

Warning!
This may be the last issue of the catalog you receive.

If we rented your name, or you haven't ordered in the last two years you may not hear from us again. If you wish to stay informed about products and services that can make a difference to your health and well-being, please indicate below.

Name ....

Address ....

City .... State ...... Zip ......

Phone ....

Do You Have A Friend Who'd Like To Receive This Catalog?

We would be happy to send your friend a free copy. Make sure to print and complete in full:

Name ....

Address ....

City .... State ...... Zip ......

DDP 04/03